GENETICS - RESEARCH AND ISSUES

DOWN SYNDROME, BEYOND THE INTELLECTUAL DISABILITY

PERSONS WITH THEIR OWN EMOTIONAL WORLD

GENETICS - RESEARCH AND ISSUES

Additional books in this series can be found on Nova's website
under the Series tab.

Additional e-books in this series can be found on Nova's website
under the e-book tab.

DISABILITY AND THE DISABLED-ISSUES, LAWS AND PROGRAMS

Additional books in this series can be found on Nova's website
under the Series tab.

Additional e-books in this series can be found on Nova's website
under the e-book tab.

GENETICS - RESEARCH AND ISSUES

DOWN SYNDROME, BEYOND THE INTELLECTUAL DISABILITY

PERSONS WITH THEIR OWN EMOTIONAL WORLD

GUADALUPE ELIZABETH MORALES

AND

ERNESTO OCTAVIO LOPEZ

NOVA BIOMEDICAL

New York

For permission to use material from this book please contact us:
Telephone 631-231-7269; Fax 631-231-8175
Web Site: http://www.novapublishers.com

Library of Congress Cataloging-in-Publication Data

ISBN: 978-1-62618-467-1

Library of Congress Control Number: 2013935454

Published by Nova Science Publishers, Inc. † New York

"To see our similarities with other people, allows us to identify ourselves and to feel we belong to a community. However, the ability to acknowledge and work with the differences we have from other people empowers our individual development as human beings."

This book is dedicated to our beloved parents Maria and Francisco, as well as Marcelino and Alice, who have filled our lives with the deepest emotions.

Contents

List of Figures

List of Tables

Preface

This book is similar to others of its kind because it provides suggestions on improvements to the quality of life for persons who have been labeled as having an intellectual disability, namely, people with Down syndrome (DS). However, this literary piece is unique and original because not only does it invite readers to better understand current modern academic knowledge related to DS and emotion theory, but it also offers new methodological keys to help drive further academic exploration into the areas of special education and DS research. By explanation of this last reason, one motivation to write many parts of the book was to diminish the painful limitations of current academic paths used to answer simple questions from parents, special education teachers and professional caregivers dealing with persons with DS.

Accordingly, the book is designed so that a newcomer to intellectual disability and DS will find chapter 1 and appendix 1 as a theoretical welcome acknowledged by many people who frequently relate to DS. In particular, updated informative descriptions are provided about the place that DS has in history, as well as its underlying genetic processes. As will be observed in chapter 1, scientific attention to Down syndrome is relatively new. It was not until 50 years ago that its etiology was discovered. Regarding psychological approaches, some advances have been made concerning the development of cognitive processes of those with this atypical genetic condition. However, whenever emotion and DS are considered together, there is still a general acknowledgment that much more exploration is needed in order to understand these dynamics inside this population, and more research is demanded. This delay in understanding the emotional lives of people with DS is mainly due to the fact that the scientific analysis of human emotion is new in general. This has contributed to the perpetuation of misconceptions about the emotional lives of this population. Introductory remarks from chapter 1 are not intended only as informative considerations, but also to promote academic scrutiny of the well-established system of misconceptions and myths regarding DS. For instance, this text brings to the reader's attention the capacity of people with DS to understand concepts like justice and morality. Misconceptions about their capacity to distinguish goodness from evil in humans is different through members inside this population, and their current civil rights do not recognize their capacity to comprehend moral, ethical and constrained justice judgment opinions. In this work, it will be emphasized that DS life improvement can be achieved by research in the academic realm, of the guidelines about how they perceive their life's significance (see also chapter 4).

Additionally, the variety of sentiments and emotions considered throughout this book, and the related topics addressed are not meant to be considered exhaustive. This work only considers positive emotions most relevant, like love and happiness, as well as the cognitive and emotional nature underlying the way those with DS conceive negativity (Chapter 4). Accordingly, in chapter 4, academic research evidence is presented that suggests we need to re-conceptualize how this population sees and feels love and happiness. By doing this, a secondary goal is to promote consciousness about improvement of their civil rights, particularly regarding their ability to have their own family and offspring. Any person who has been related directly or indirectly to persons with DS will easily recognize that for an adult person with DS to love someone else inside or outside is a most profound matter that empowers them to find significance in their lives. As it will be discussed, the capacity to love another person among their own group varies, and law regulations currently do not address their need to express love. In this sense, much of the scientific evidence presented regarding DS in emotion research, rely on existing beliefs about people with DS's emotional capacities. Society is in debt to these "eternal happy children" and we would do well to re-conceptualize life the way they see it; nature it may have found another way to express itself. In some instances, at least the authors of this book believe, we can and should learn from them.

In addition to the reasons stated above for reading, those who are acquainted with scientific exploration will find some refreshing and original ideas on how to import powerful and rigorous experimental methods from other scientific fields to exceed previous limitations to explore the emotion system of people with DS's. Specifically, cognitive science methodology related to emotion theory like affective priming, connectionist neuro-computational simulations, information integration theory (cognitive algebra), and other cognitive methodological considerations, are brought into chapters 2, 3, 4 to envision as never before how is it that people with DS perceive negative elements from their social context, and how they conceptualize their sentimental life, and the concept of justice. However, since this book intends to assist a wide variety of readers (special education teachers, caregivers and parents alike), these methodological considerations are frequently presented in a simplified manner. Well-versed academic researchers are invited to read the suggested readings for additional and more technical study. This book's methodological proposal is to motivate a new generation of scientists with new points of view, to push past current analysis of research challenges in special education. It is our strong conviction that the research tools and experimental paradigms to achieve new goals are now available.

Finally, a book like this cannot be the result of a solitary effort. We are incredibly thankful for the support we have had over the past years from many people and institutions, such as CONACYT, who provided their assistance (project No. 181622). We are also thankful to people with DS from the Down Institute from Monterrey, The Down Institute from Cuernavaca, the Special Education Public Secretariat from Nuevo Leon, Mexico and other special education institutions like CAMs of Victoria City (Tamaulipas, Mexico). Their desire to improve social conditions and personal quality of life for people with DS is remarkable, and has ingrained upon us an unforgettable experience. They inspire us to continue.

Chapter 1

Down Syndrome: Beyond a Genetic Condition Linked to Intellectual Disability

Abstract

It is estimated that over 6 million people live with a small genetic variation called Down syndrome (DS) (Down syndrome Research and Treatment foundation, 2012). While the majority of books reporting this syndrome categorize this genetic condition under physical and intellectual disability (ID), it is our strongest belief that DS can be better conceptualized via a richer and wider perspective. For instance, this condition can teach us another way to experience human life. Thus, although there are not too many academic reports on the way members of this population conceptualize or find significance in their life, the writers of this book have put an enormous effort into compiling scarce academic resources in order to present coordinated and insightful ideas about how those with DS percieve their lives, in particular their emotional lives. In doing so, new academic suggestions as to how to explore the DS' emotional world will be introduced. At the same time a strong call is made for psychological research into DS exploration, which lags far behind other fields, because of the insights it may offer to this population and to the ID field in general.

As we will discuss over the following chapters, emotion, theory and DS can be a watershed to academic research because the genetically constrained DS emotional system allows us to explore the unique controlled and automatic complex cognitive and emotional processes that occur when our emotional system is experiencing atypical brain conditions. We will also be presenting evidence that, psychologically speaking, people with DS are not all the same. Improvements to their quality of life, including civil rights, can be achieved through recognition of what this study suggests. In particular, knowing more about how and why these people perceive their life as they do, supports enacting of guidelines against discrimination and corrects false stereotypes regarding DS which have been created from historical misperceptions. Let us expand the concepts by beginning with a review of how DS was historically considered, its etiology, as well as a brief introduction on psychological considerations of people with DS.

1.1. Am I Equal or Different?

In regard to the question above, let us begin with a segment of an interview with the father (Mr. Javier) of a young teenager with DS (Sophie), since some interesting commentary can be found:

> "When I am at the mall with her I do realize people notice her, but most of the time she will not recognize herself as having a handicap. Indeed she will not, and frequently my daughter will assert, "I AM EQUAL TO EVERYBODY". However, when a famous artist came to town, she tried to enter the star's dressing room, but security did not permit her to pass. She then began shouting "LET ME ENTER, I AM A DOWN SYNDROME GIRL, I AM SPECIAL". She was using every ability she possessed to enter the place. From my personal point of view, she has a lot of ability. She is a COMMON person whenever it is convenient to her but also she is a DOWN SYNDROME person whenever it is necessary to be. This pleases me because trying to achieve something we want is a NATURAL ABILITY OF HUMAN BEINGS."

Mr. Javier's words encompass at least three considerations relevant to scientific psychology: a) The capacity of a person to establish regularities (I AM EQUAL TO EVERYBODY), b) the acknowledgment of human variety (LET ME ENTER, I AM A DOWN SYNDROME GIRL, I AM SPECIAL) and c) adaptive social behaviour (NATURAL ABILITY OF HUMAN BEINGS). Furthermore, the described scenario displays the person's desire for group belongingness and connected desire to ensure no loss of individuality occurs. Both conditions are necessary for proper human development. On the other hand, Sophie has displayed one of Darwin's premises regarding evolution, which is survival through adaptation to a hostile social context. She has learnt to use her genetic condition to differentiate herself from others. As we will discuss in the next several chapters, this self-perception originates in a complex cognitive and emotional way to perceive the world. As we will see later this self-perception relates to DS variability and the social circumstances that surround it.

1.2. Down Syndrome: Another Color in the Human Rainbow Spectrum

Human nature expresses itself differently in each of us. If you look at each member of your family, you notice how different each is via behaviour, personality, tastes, etc. If it were not for physical similarities, it might even be difficult to say the members belong to the same family. Human differences are connected to a wide range of origins and forms, and are frequently hard to classify. Even so, Figure 1.1. shows how differences might be classified (see The Linux Information Project, 2005).

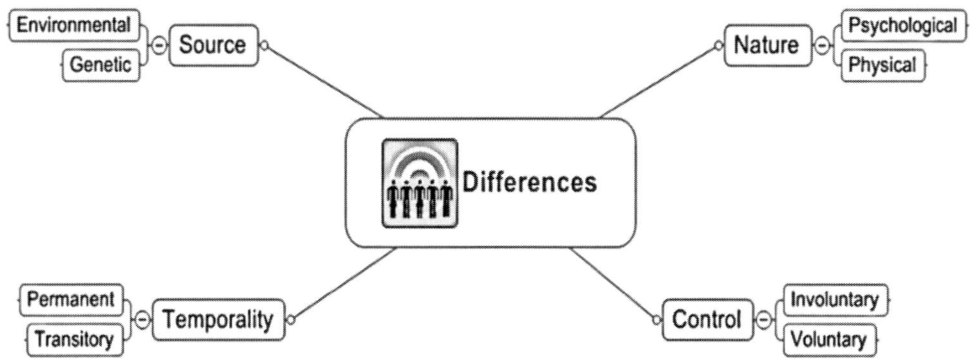

Figure 1.1. A simple graph of how human diversity might be classified through different criteria.

Human variation enhances our everyday life and it empowers improvement. However, this human characteristic has not always had a positive connotation. For instance, in the early 1800s biological variation was conceived as a synonym of impurity, similar to the concept of inorganic mineral impurity (Roughgarden, 2004). This negative connotation has had a tremendous impact on the history of society, and methods to control this "impurity" have led to well-documented historical cases of genocide or extermination of individuals based on physical or intellectual ideals (see Schleichkorn, 1981; Morales, Lopez, Charles, Castro & Sanchez, 2013). Thus, the concept of "being different" has since ancestral times implied a rejection, something to be feared or denoted a target for cruelty. Even in our time, it is common to see how this system of beliefs against natural variation unleashes irrational discrimination.

A non-biased initial characterization of human variation can be defined as a set of possible physical and psychological values or states a human can assume. In terms of physical attributes, one may consider a wide spectrum of observable values, like weight, height, etc., whereas psychologically speaking, nonphysical variables (such as cognitive processing operations, mental activity states) and observable characteristics like attitude, temper, creativity, moral virtue, etc. characterise a good portrait of a human being. Variations in these human values may occur systematically as well as randomly, and comprise different affection intensity over our life span. For instance, biologically speaking, around 750 atypical genetic variations (among them, Prader-Willi syndrome, Fragile X syndrome, Down syndrome, etc.) have been identified as systematically affecting the cognitive and behavioural capacity of the human beings who have these conditions (Hodapp, DesJardin & Ricci, 2003). However, these biological constraints are not by themselves the reason for discrimination, cruelty or rejection, but rather because of an existing system of misconceptions about the human manifestation, due to physiological affectations.

In this sense, it is important to support systematic efforts to improve living conditions for people with intellectual disabilities (ID), including how to re-conceptualize misconceptions about these genetic conditions and their human manifestations. Take for instance the effort to change a previous myth that ID is inherent and inseparable from what a person is (e.g. "a mental retard"), toward the concept of someone with a different life condition (e.g. "a person with ID"). This re-conceptualization process is necessary to understand DS, and throughout this book, academic notes will be introduced to this end. Let us for the moment simply note that this syndrome was once conceptualized as a form of sickness, thus the main consideration consisted of medical diagnosis and possible treatments. This medical portrait was blended with a portrait of personal and human characteristics that typify members of this population, which led to non-favorable social conditions, including segregation / ostracism.

Fortunately, beliefs regarding DS have gradually changed from that of a sickness-based portrait to that of a view of it as a life condition. Several reasons may account for this change, among them, life expectancy. Since members of this population have increased their life expectancy, there is an increased interest to integrating them as productive members of a society. This is possible with a new academic understanding of their intellectual, social and emotional functioning.

1.3. A Different Genetic Path that Leads to the Same Place: A Human Being

Just to clarify the intended meaning of the DS genetic condition, let us introduce some brief genetic concepts underlying this syndrome (a more extensive description is presented in Appendix 1).

Every cell in our body (billions of them) contains within its nucleus a set of chromosomes, or "packages", built from proteins and DNA (Deoxyribonucleic acid). These pre-packed molecules have codified information about how to build a human. Most of us have 46 chromosomes (in 23 chromosome pairs) in each of our cells, but some persons may have more, or fewer. While the genetic result of chromosome variation is always still a "human being", chromosomal variation has a tremendous impact upon a person's quality of life. This is the case for people with DS; members of this population are born with a third instance of chromosome 21 (or an additional partial chromosome 21). This genetic variation has a profound effect on physical development (e.g., weight, facial displays, hands with different physical appearances, etc.), health (increased probability of cardiac arrest), and, as we will discuss in later chapters, a systemic effect upon cognitive and emotional architecture.

1.3.1. Down Syndrome: Definition and Origins

As we have mentioned, the Down syndrome (DS) is a genetic condition caused by the presence of an additional chromosome 21 in the cells of a person. Currently, this chromosome variation is one of the most commonly reported. Estimated occurrence for this syndrome in the world population is about 1 per each 800 living newborns, that is, every year, around 150,000 newborn babies with DS are welcomed in our world (Basile, 2008; Irvine, 2007; Kingston 2002; Lambert & Rondal, 1989; Roizen & Patterson, 2003; Sadler, 2004; Stratford, 1998; Lubec, 2003; Roizen & Patterson, 2003; Santos & Morizon, 1999; Sanz, Salguero, Cásanovas, Holanda & Vivas, 2000).

Although there is no precise first historical record of this genetic condition, paintings, as well as some anthropological evidence, suggest its presence in our ancestors. For example, curious but intriguing academic speculation has suggested that the almost 3000-year-old stone-cut Mexican Olmeca heads might be facial representations of DS individuals (Stratford, 1998). These stone faces contain many of the particular characteristics of a face with DS, and Olmecas might have decided to build them because they believed that sacred people were characterized by unusual physical abnormalities or unusual mental states (Guerrero, 1995; Stratford, 1988). A less speculative anthropological record is the finding of a Saxon skull from the age of VII A.D. The cranium possesses all the structural characteristics that define a DS head (Lopez, Lopez, Pares, Borges & Valdespino, 2000).

Furthermore, inside the artistic field, some paintings from the 15th and 18th centuries have attracted academic attention due to their representations of people with DS. Such is the case of the painting titled "The Virgin and the Andrea Mantegna Child" (1430-1506), as well as the Sir Joshua Reynolds' painting (1723-1792) entitled "Lady Cockburn and Her Children", both of which display a child with DS characteristics (Pueschel, 2001; Straford, 1998).

In addition to these first possible visual historical records of DS existence, formal written reports detailing aspects of this genetic condition can be found which date back to the 19th century (Pueschel, 2001). Among these reports is the first medical analysis written by Esquirol in 1838, followed by a detailed written description of Seguin in 1846, who named this genetic condition as *idiocia furfuracea*. Additional contributions can be found in Duncans' description (1866) of a little girl with DS, and in John Langdon's academic paper entitled, "*Observations on an ethnic classification of idiots*", published by the *London Hospital Clinical Lectures and Reports* in 1866. Thanks to this paper, John Langdon is known as the discoverer and creator of the first detailed clinical analysis of the DS genetic condition (Irvine, 2007; Jay, 1999; Lopez et al., 2000).

For his part, Down (1866) believed that most intellectual disabilities were due to variances in the human race. Specifically, he believed, based on personal observations, that physical attributes from the Mongol race were also present in DS. Because of this, he initially called this genetic condition Mongolic idiocy. However, due to concerns about being politically incorrect, different authors proposed different academic terms like *acromicria* or *peristaltic amnesia* to classify the condition (Stratford, 1998). Finally in 1961, a team of scientists (among them a relative of Dr. Down) proposed describing the genetic condition by its current name. The World Health Organization (WHO) in 1965 changed the nomenclature to Down syndrome after a formal request by the Mongolian government (Howard-Jones, 1979; Patterson & Costa, 2005).

From its initial diagnosis to the present, there has been a noticeable and growing interest in enhancing our understanding of DS in various academic fields. There is no doubt that a major advance in understanding DS was the discovery of the genetic mechanism underlying the condition, by Dr. Lejuene in 1959. From that point, insights regarding possible genetic mechanisms leading to DS have been proposed, and because of their relevance, these are discussed next, in order to frame the different levels of understanding that are required where a person with DS is concerned.

1.3.2. Down Syndrome Etiology and Classification

More than a century of intense academic research on the etiology of DS has passed since its first clinical description. Many of the initial theoretical models were highly speculative and nonsystematic. Take for instance Dr. Down (1866) who, with contemporary colleagues, argued that DS was related to tuberculosis, since parents of this population had a history of having such a sickness. Other explanatory approaches to DS (see Table 1.1.) linked it to syphilis, alcoholism, endocrine dysfunction, environmental factors during pregnancy, uterus tiredness, parents' age, etc. (Patterson & Costa, 2005). Through time, most of these hypotheses were either partially or completely discarded. Even so, it is relevant to emphasize that the effects these academic views had over the general population perception of people with DS has remained to the present, and specifically, those views linking race to DS.

Table 1.1. Some etiology theories about Down syndrome

Theory	Some antecedents	Principal postulate
Dishonor theory	Sutherland's paper (1899) entitled *Mongolian imbecility in infants* suggested that DS was caused by syphilis. Cafferata published *Contribution a la literature du mongolisme* in 1909, where he proposed that parental alcoholism was the cause for trisomy 21.	These theories proposed that DS was due to dishonorable behaviours as alcholism or promiscuous sexual activities.
Crookshank Atavism race theory	Down (1866), in his paper *Observations on an ethnic classification of idiots* described the characteristics of DS and related them to physical attributes of Mongol people. In 1924 Crookshank published *The Mongol in Our Midst* where he presented his atavism theory.	Crookshank's theory assumed that DS was a regression towards a more primitive race.
Endocrine-based Theories	Clark and Edin (1928) wrote in their article *The mongol: a new explanation* that DS was due to endocrine imbalance that had its origins in a probable hiperthyroidism from the mother, thus suggesting that excessive thyroidism secretions during pregnancy have a negative impact over the fetus' development. Some other theoretical speculations pointed to the absence of internal organ strength and glandular dysfunction in the child (Guerrero, 1995).	Either parents or their child had an endocrine inbalance that led to DS.
Family factors Theories	Shuttleworth in 1909 suggested for the very first time that a mature mothers' age might be a risk factor.	Parents' age as the main reason to develop DS.

Although initial etiology models of DS did not approach a diagnosis of this condition from a genetic point of view, it was implicit since the beginning of the 20th century that a chromosomal mechanism could be the main factor. It was not until 1930 that some researchers began to propose that this condition might be a chromosome-based problem. Specifically, Waardenburg (1932) suggested that this syndrome was related either to chromosome duplication or to the absence of one or more chromosomes. On his part, Bleyer (1934) proposed that unequal chromosome migration was the cause. Interestingly, Turpin (1937), Southwick (1939) and Penrose (1939) (cited by Carter, 2002), also suggested a chromosome variance, but they did not refer to it as a dysfunction.

It was hard to discard any of these initial genetic approaches due to the fact that genetic identification technology at that time was not sophisticated enough to allow for chromosome counting. In 1956, however, Dr. Tijo and Dr. Levan were able to identify the exact number of chromosomes in human cells. This major breakthrough in genetics led to Lejeune, Gautier & Trupin (1959a, 1959b) investigating, and identifying the existence of an extra chromosome inside the cells of people with DS. Specifically, in two different research studies, they showed the existence of 47 chromosomes in Down syndrome cells, in contrast to the 46 chromosomes found by Tijo and Levan inside the cells of typical individuals. Leujene et al. argued that the chromosome variance was due to a non-disjunction (non-separation) of a chromosome pair during the cell meiosis process; specifically in chromosome 21.

Further scientific research from independent studies confirmed this genetic finding (e.g., Jacobs, Baikie, Court-Brown & Strong, 1959). These academic findings led to the identification and classification of this genetic condition as trisomy 21. The primary cause for this trisomy remains unknown; however there is a precise genetic characterization of the genetic mechanisms underlying the condition (for details see Appendix 1). For example, it is known that a chromosome non-disjunction occurs during the cell division process (Stratford, 1998). Depending on when this genetic distribution error occurs, different forms of DS can occur. More specifically, the time at which chromosome distribution appears determines the severity and quality (e.g. mosaic DS; Pimentel & Dyce, 2003) of the clinical manifestations of the syndrome. At the time of writing, three different classifications for this syndrome are known: Regular trisomy 21, mosaic DS and DS translocation.

Regular trisomy 21 implies the existence of an extra chromosome in the 21 pair of every cell. This genetic condition is the most frequent in DS. It is calculated that between 80 to 95 percent of people with DS are characterized by trisomy 21 (Guerrero, 1995; Jasso, 1991; Lambert & Rondal, 1989; Sadler, 2004; Stratford 1998). It is unknown why regular trisomy 21 occurs, but it is argued that the condition appears at random. There are also genetic scenarios wherein only a small portion of the cell's body presents an extra 21 chromosome, while the rest have the typical genetic structure. This condition is known as mosaic DS (Jasso, 1991; Lambert & Rondal, 1989; Stratford, 1998). This genetic condition is hard to detect because is rare. It is estimated that incidence of this condition occurs between 1 to 2 percent of the population with DS (Basile, 2008). The last DS kind we will refer to is known as translocation. This phenomenon occurs whenever a part or the whole of a chromosome combines with another one. In these situations, chromosome 21 blends with other chromosome pairs such as chromosomes 13, 14 or 15 (Jasso, 1991), and possibly, links to itself or to chromosome 22 (Kingston, 2002). This genetic condition represents almost 5% of the cases, and occurs spontaneously during the first cellular division. Parents affected by this syndrome will pass it on to their offspring (Jasso, 1991; Kingston, 2002; Stratford, 1998).

Academic researchers involved in genetics suggest that is important to identify the kind of chromosome distribution error as well as the chromosome localization and extension, because this information is related to determining the severity of DS (see Patterson & Costa, 2005).

Hodapp et al. (2003) argues that intellectual disability etiology is not only typified by medical-physical characterization; there are also behavioural phenotypes related to the syndrome that are relevant in determining the person's life span. This seems to be the case for people with DS who not only present physical and medical characteristics that differentiate them from typical people, but also present specific psychological and behavioural conditions. Some of these will be discussed next.

1.4. Down Syndrome Phenotype: Unique, Equal, or Special?

One major concern for people with DS who wish to be included in society is the eradication of discrimination against them. This monumental task has created heated debates on how those with DS may differ from the general population in terms of cognitive, emotional and behavioural displays. Misconceptions lead to assignment of inaccurate stereotypes, and it is for this reason that a well-defined phenotype is so needed. Such a DS phenotype will allow to correctly frame the syndrome (Korenberg, Chen, Schipper, Sun, Gonsky, Gerwehr, Yamanaka, 1994), and also permit proper clinical diagnosis and intervention (Antonarakis & Epstein, 2006, abstract) as well as widen our understanding of how genetic variation affects human life (Antonarakis, Lyle, Dermitzakis, Reymond, & Deutsch, 2004).

Currently, very few are willing talk in terms of *differences due to genetic conditions* since there is a fear—not unfounded—that such discussion may promote stereotypes that lead to discrimination. Also, since there is a wide swath of possible phenotype manifestations to DS (Roper & Reeves, 2006), disagreement remains over what would be called specific DS phenotype traits, since there is no assurance they are exclusive, dependent or characteristic of only this syndrome (Fidler, 2005). For instance some traits appear only on some members with DS and not on the rest of their population (Antonarakis et al., 2004). Even those traits that have a high probability of appearing throughout the population with DS seem to vary in expression. Consider as just one example, how intellectual disability varies from low to high inside the DS population (e.g., Patterson, 2007).

The phenotype of a syndrome includes different physical and psychological aspects from a person (e.g. cognitive, behavioural and emotional). It can be simply defined as the probability of a person having some specific traits during development that are not presented by individuals who do not have the syndrome (Dykens, 1995).

Table 1.2. Some of the most frequent signs related to the Down syndrome phenotype

Down Syndrome physical and psychological characteristics				
Physical	**Neural**	**Cognitive**	**Behavioural**	**Emotional**
• Small head • Thin hair • Almond-shaped eyes • Droopy eyelids • Flat and short nose • Large tongue • A short and wide neck • Small ears as well as short teeth and hands • Short extremities • Overweight • Bruised skin • Hypotonia	• Pathological Neurochemistry • Progressive Neurochemistry changes	• Intellectual disability (from low to high). • Information processing difficulties • Low attention focus • Declarative memory problems • Difficulties for memory coding and retrieval • Echoic memory difficulties • Better performance for visual memory tasks • High probability of developing Alzheimer disease between the ages of 40 and 50	• They present more inappropiate behaviour than typical individuals. • However, they do present less non-adaptive behaviour than other intelectual discapacity populations.	• Slow emotional development. • High chance of developing depression at later age • Increased probability of developing anxiety

1.4.1. Some Final Remarks on DS and Its Definitory Characteristics

Some empirical data suggests that DS systematically constrains cognitive, emotional and behavioural development (see Table 1.2).

At the physical level, there are commonly observed salient facial and body attributes. Some initial descriptions of this physical phenotype can be found even before the syndrome had been formally described. For example, Duncan (1866, p.35) provided a description of what seems to be a child with DS: "A female child, aged twelve years; has a small head with a high sugar-loaf shape, Chinese-looking eyes, and a long projecting lower lip. The face is very plain…". The same year, Dr. Down presented one of the first clinical descriptions of the syndrome that included physical descriptions of patients with trisomy 21 as follows:

> "The hair is not truly black like the one of the Mongol people, it is more like non-abundant, dark brown, straight hair. Their face is rather plain and wide, with no prominent features. The face also has rounded cheeks, laterally extended. Their eyes are turned and their lips are thick, with transversal fissures. In addition, the tongue is large, wide and rough. The nose is short and the skin has a yellowish tint…."

Many physical attributes noted by Down in 1866 remain valid descriptions of the modern DS phenotype. However, references to ethnic characteristics have been discarded due to racist connnotations. At present, at least 50 physical and psychological characteristics are used to frame DS. Table 1.2 shows the most frequent traits used by researchers (e.g., Basile, 2008; Chapman & Hesketh, 2000; Dyknes, 1995; Loeches et al., 1991) and DS institutions (e.g., National Dissemination Center for Children with Disabilities, 2004). It is important to note that not all members in the DS population manifest every phenotype attribute. Group variance is present, just as occurs in the general population even when the phenotype assumes homogeneity (Chapman & Hesketh, 2000). Social context, family factors as well as individual differences (like personality) contribute to this, within variance, from very early ontogeny and through all the developmental stages of a person with DS.

In addition to the above DS phenotype specifications, members of this population have higher probability of presenting congenital problems (e.g. congenital heart disease problems as well as severe gastrointestinal problems), endocrine problems, and hematologic, ophthalmic, orthopedic, psychiatric, gynecologic problems as well, among others (Basile, 2008; Loeches et al., 1991; Santos & Morizon, 1999).

Regarding people with DS development it is not clear if these problems should be defined in terms of that presented by a typical individual with the difference being they're typical but in slow motion (Wishart, 2001). What is known is that the cognitive performance spectrum varies from almost typical to severe intellectual disability (Basile, 2008; Sroufe, 1998). Generally speaking the IQ (intellectual quotient) levels in this population tend to range from 36 to 107, with scores declining around the age of 40 years old (Roizen & Patterson, 2003; Wang, 1996). Regarding this, Loeches et al. (1991), has identified some research trends that relate the DS phenotype within variance (regular, mosaic or translocation) and IQ variance in this population. However, the link between cognitive function and the syndrome remains undiscovered since there is no conclusive empirical corpus to support one. Even so, since mosaic DS shows more genotype and phenotype heterogeneity than other genetic scenarios in the same syndrome, it is expected to link to more IQ score variability and other psychological differences. Generally speaking, it seems that intellectual development inside this group seems to follow a cognitive developmental pattern similar to typical individuals, but in slow motion or seemingly paused (Lambert & Rondal, 1989). In addition, people with DS display language deficits and short term memory difficulties.

There are bigger debates when it comes to defining a phenotype for personality, behavioural and emotional factors, because of doubts on how precise a phenotype can be, and what methods should be considered to define a specific trait (Flint, 1998).

It is important to note that the DS population does present fewer difficulties in terms of behavioural problems and adaptation compared to other populations with an intellectual disability (Chapman & Hesketh, 2000; Fidler, Hodapp & Dykens, 2002). In contrast, some authors argue that people with DS tend to demand more attention; they seem to present more stubbornness and disobedience than typical individuals (e.g. Pueschel, Bernier & Pezzullo, 1991). Relevant to this atypical behavioural repertoire is their emotional behaviour, which seems highly constrained by the underlying genetic condition (e.g. Carvajal & Iglesias, 2000; Kasari, Freeman & Bass, 2003; Sroufe, 1998). As will be addressed in next chapter, defining this emotional behaviour as a "deficit" is highly controversial, as well as misleading.

1.5. Recapping Some Ideas

Similarity and diversity are part of human nature. People, even if they belong to different groups, intersect in several aspects maintaining their personal identity that makes them different. Figure 1.2 shows graphically this idea regarding DS and group with typical development.

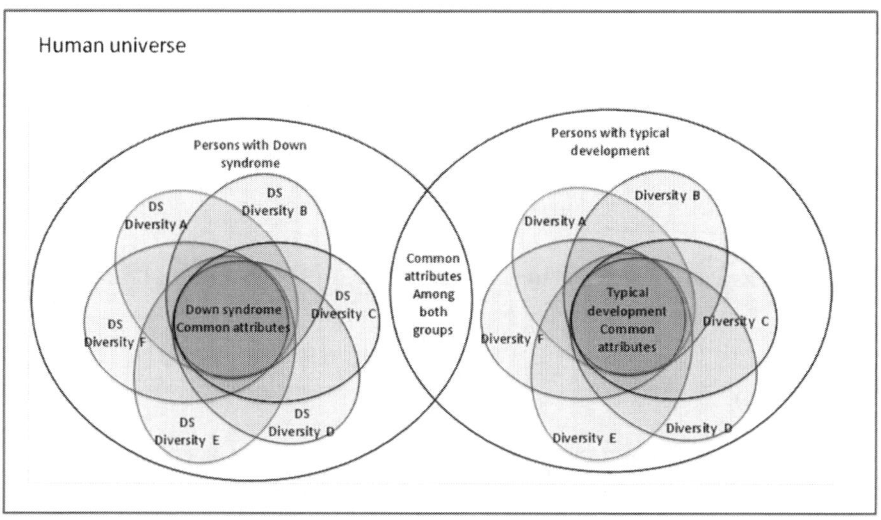

Figure 1.2. Graphical representation of communality and variability between these two groups (people with typical development versus Down syndrome). Communality and variability can be observed inside of each group.

Regarding Figure 1.2, the goal of DS science is to predict and exactly determine intersection percentages as well as percentage differences among the different biological and psychological attributes typifying the DS population. This book represents an invitation to look forward by considering current methods and theory from the cognitive science of emotion field. By comprehending more on such variability it is assumed that the characteristics misapplied to this genetically constrained population will be finally acknowledged.

References

Antonarakis, S. E., Lyle, R., Dermitzakis, E. T., Reymond, A. & Deutsch, S. (2004). Chromosome 21 and Down syndrome: from genomics to pathophysiology. *Nature Reviews*, 5, 725–738.

Antonarakis, S. E. & Epstein, C. J. (2006). The challenge of Down syndrome. *Trends in Molecular Medicine, 12*(10), 473–479. doi: http://dx.doi.org/10.1016/j.bbr.2011.03.031

Basile, H. (2008). Retraso mental y genética: Síndrome de Down. *Alcmeon, Revista Argentina de Clínica Neuropsiquiatrica, Año XVII, 15*(1), 9-23.

Bleyer, A. (1934). Indications that mongoloid idiocy is a gametic mutation of degenerative type. *American Journal of Diseases of Children*, *47*, 342-48

Cafferata, J. F. (1909). Contribution a la literature du mongolisme. *Arch Med Enf, 12*, 929.

Carter, K. C. (2002). Early Conjectures That Down syndrome is caused by chromosomal nondisjunction. *Bulletin of the History of Medicine, 76*(3), 528-563.

Carvajal, F. & Iglesias, J. (2000). Looking behaviour and smiling in Down syndrome infants. *Journal of Nonverbal Behaviour*, *24*(3), 225-236.

Chapman, R. S. & Hesketh, L. J. (2000). Behavioural phenotype of individuals with Down syndrome. *Mental Retardation and Developmental Disabilities Research Reviews, 6*(2), 84-95.

Clark, R. M. & Edin, M. B. (1928). The mongol: a new explanation. *Journal of Mental Science, 74,* 739-747.

Crookshank, F. G. (1924). *In The Mongol in our Midst*. London: Kegan Paul, Trench and Trubner Ltd.

Down, J. L. (1866). Observations on ethnic classification of idiots. *London Hospital. Clinical Lectures and Reports, 3,*259-262.

Down Syndrome Research and Treatment Foundation (n/d). DS 101. Retrieved January 30, 2012 from http://www.dsrtf.org/page.aspx?pid=352

Duncan, P. & Millard, W. (1866). *A Manual for the Classification Training, and Education of the Feeble-minded, imbecile and idiotic*. London: Longmans, Green.

Dykens, E. M. (1995). Measuring behavioural phenotypes: Provocations from "the new genetics". *American Journal of Mental Retardation, 99*(5), 522-532.

Esquirol, J. (1838). *Des maladies mentales considerees sous les rapports medical, hygienique et medico-legal*. Paris: Baillière, ed.

Fidler, D. J. (2005). The emerging Down syndrome behavioural phenotype in early childhood. *Infants & Young Children,* 18(2), 86–103.

Fidler, D., Hodapp, R. & Dykens, E. (2002). Behavioural phenotypes and special education: parent report of educational issues for children with Down syndrome, Prader-Willi syndrome and Williams syndrome. *The Journal of Special Education, 36*(2), 80-88.

Flint, J. (1998). al phenotypes: conceptual and methodological Issues. American Journal of Medical Genetics (Neuropsychiatric Genetics), 81, 235–240.

Guerrero, L. J. (1995). *Nuevas perspectivas en la educación e integración de los niños con síndrome de Down*. México: Paidós.

Hodapp, R. M. (2001). Etiology and personality-motivation: Direct and indirect effects. In H. Switzky (Ed.), Motivation and self-system processes in mental retardation (pp. 257-282). Hillsdale, NJ: Erlbaum

Hodapp, R. M., DesJardin, J. L. & Ricci, L. A. (2003). Genetic syndromes of mental retardation: should they matter for the early interventionist? *Infants and Young Children, 16*(2), 152-160.

Howard-Jones, N. (1979). On the diagnostic term Down's disease. *Medical History, 23*(1), 102-104.

Irvine, P. (2007). Down, J. (John) Langdon (1828-1896). In C. R. Reynolds & Fletcher-Janzen (Eds.). Encyclopedia of special education: a reference for the education of children adolescents and adults with disabilities and other exceptional individuals (Vol. 1, pp. 760). NJ, EE. UU.: John Wiley & Sons.

Jacobs, P. A., Baikie A. G., Court-Brown, W. M., Strong, J. A. (1959). The somatic chromosomes in mongolism. *Lancet, 1*(7075), 710.

Jasso, L. (1991). *El niños Down: mitos y realidades*. Mexico, D.F.: Manual Moderno.

Jay, V. (1999). Dr. John Langdon Down. *Archives of Pathology & Laboratory Medicine, 123*(2), 102

Kasari, C., Freeman, S. F. & Bass, W. (2003). Empathy and response to distress in children with Down syndrome. *Journal of Child Psychology and Psychiatry, 44*(3), 424-431.

Kingston, H. (2002). *ABC of clinical genetics*. Londres: BMJ.

Korenberg, J. R., Chen, X.-N., Schipper, R., Sun, Z., Gonsky, R., Gerwehr, S. & Yamanaka, T. (1994). Down syndrome phenotypes: The consequences of chromosomal imbalance. *Proc. Nati. Acad. Sci., 91*, 4997-5001.

Lambert, J. & Rondal, J. (1989). *El mongolismo*. Barcelona: Herder.

Lejeune, J. (1959). Le mongolism: premier exemple d'aberration autosomique humaine. *Ann Genet, 1*, 41–49.

Lejeune, J., Gauthier, M. & Turpin, R. (1959a). Les chromosomes humains en culture de tissus. *Comptes Rendus de l'Academie des Sciences, 248*, 602-603.

Lejeune, J., Gauthier, M. & Turpin, R. (1959b). Etudes des chromosomes somatiques de neuf enfants mongoliens. *Comptes Rendus de l'Academie des Sciences,* 248, 1721-1722

Loeches, A. A., Iglesias, D. J. & Carvajal, M. F. (1991) Psicobiología del síndrome de Down. *Aprendizaje, Estudios de Psicología, 46,* 107-128.

Lopez, P., Lopez, R., Páres, G., Borges, A. & Valdespino, L (2000). Reseña histórica del síndrome Down. *ADM LVII*, (5), 193-199.

Lubec, G. (2003). *The brain in Down syndrome (trisomy 21)*. Recuperado el 13 de abril de 2004, de http://www.altonweb.com/cs/downsyndrome/lubec.html.

Morales, G. E., Lopez, R. E. Charles, D. J. Castro, C. & Sanchez, M. P. (2013). *Parental and educators' judgments and attitudes toward life challenges of persons with intellectual disability: Functional measurement contributions to special education from a cognitive algebra approach.* USA: NOVA Science Publisher.

National Dissemination Center for Children with Disabilities (2010). *Discapacidades Intelectuales* [Intellectual disabilities]. Retrieved November 20, 2012, from http://nichcy.org/wp-content/uploads/docs/spanish/fs8sp.pdf

Patterson, D. & Costa, A. C. S. (2005). History of genetic disease: Down syndrome and genetics a case of linked histories. *Nature Reviews Genetics, 6*(2), 137-147.

Patterson, D. (2007). Genetic mechanisms involved in the phenotype of Down syndrome. *Mental Retardation and Developmental Disabilities, Research Reviews*, 13, 199 – 206.

Pimentel, B. H. & Dyce, G. B. (2003). Caracterización citogenética del síndrome de Down. *Revista Medica Internacional sobre el Síndrome Down*. Recuperado el 15 de noviembre de 2003, de http://www.fcsd.org/cas/revista/suscriptores.html

Pueschel, S. M. (2001). *A parent's guide to Down syndrome: Toward a brighter future* (2a. ed.). EE. UU.: Paul H. Brookes Publishing Co.

Pueschel, S. M., Bernier, J. C. & Pezzullo, J. C. (1991). Behavioural observations in children with Down's syndrome. *Journal of Intellectual Disability Research*, 35(6), 502-511.

Roizen, N. & Patterson, D. (2003). Down's syndrome. *The lancet, 361*(9365), 1281-1289.

Roper, R. J. & Reeves, R. H. (2006). Understanding the basis for Down syndrome phenotypes. *PLoS Genetics, 2*(3), 231-236. doi: 10.1371/journal.pgen.0020050

Roughgarden, J. (2004). *Evolution's rainbow: diversity, gender and sexuality in nature and people*. Berkeley: University of California Press

Sadler, T. W. (2004). *Embriología médica: con orientación clínica* (10a. ed.) México: Médica Panamericana.

Stratford, B. (1998). *Síndrome de Down: pasado, presente y futuro*. México: Edivision.

Santos, M. J. & Morizon, G. (1999). Enfoque clínico del síndrome de Down. *Pediatría al día, 15*(1), 29-33.

Sanz, E., Salguero, Cásanovas, V., Holanda, M. & Vivas, L. M. (2000). *Historia del síndrome Down*. C.E.S. Madrid: Universidad Complutense.

Schleichkorn, J. (1981). Deinstitutionalization and Normalization of Persons with Mental Retardation: The Role of a Physical Therapist in Community Placement. *Journal of the American Physical Therapy Association. 61*(10), 1438-1441.

Sroufe, A. (1998). *Desarrollo emocional: la organización de la vida emocional en los primeros años*. México, D.F.: Oxford University Press.

Stratford, B. (1998). *Síndrome de Down: pasado, presente y futuro*. México: Edivision.

Sutherland, G. A. (1899). Mongolian imbecility in infants. *Practitioner, 63*, 632.

Shuttleworth G. E.(1909). Mongolian imbecility. *British Medical Journal, 2,* 661–5

The Linux Information Project (2005). *Human variability: A brief Introduction*. Retrieved April 17, 2012, from http://www.linfo.org/human_variability.html

Tijo, J. H. & Levan A. (1956). The chromosome number of man. *Hereditas*, 42, 1-6. Retrieved January 02, 2013, from http://digital.csic.es/bitstream/10261/15776/1/TjioJH_Hereditas_1956.pdf

Waardenburg, P. J. (1932). In *das menschliche auge und seine erbalagen*. Haag: Martinus Nijhoff.

Wang, P. P. (1996). A neuropsychological profile of Down syndrome: Cognitive skills and brain morphology. *Mental Retardation and Developmental Disabilities Research Reviews, 2*(2), 102-108.

Wishart, J. (2001). Motivation and learning styles in young children with Down syndrome. *Down Syndrome Research and Practice, 7*(2), 47-51. doi: 10.3104/reports.113

World Health Organization (2001). *International classification of functioning, disability, and health (ICF).* Geneva: Author. Retrieved November 20, 2012, from http://www.disabilitaincifre.it/documenti/ICF_18.pdf

Chapter 2

Do Persons with Down Syndrome Have a Divergent Emotional Mind?

Abstract

The emotional mind of persons with Down syndrome (DS) is a fascinating and unknown field for psychology. As it will be argued next, enhancing our scientific understanding of the way a person with DS emotionally signifies the world will be one of the most relevant challenges in next decades. In this chapter, our main objective is to present a very general overview on what is known about the emotional world of those with DS. Different aspects of their emotional behaviour, regulation, perception and experience are briefly reviewed using current emotion theory.

2.1. Down Syndrome as a Window to Understand Human Emotional Nature

One day, the mother of a young person with DS told us:

> "My son and I used to walk every day by the same places in our house. One day my husband and I gave him a present… a camera. That day, he walked again with me by the usual places, and he suddenly stopped in front of an ornament that for me has no meaning. However, he took a picture of this object, so now I can perceive his way of seeing things. He has an almost artistic sense of things; he transforms simple objects into the most beautiful things".

Persons with DS are commonly described as people skilled at perceiving and transforming little details into strong emotional expressions; it is as if they are artists of emotion. In accordance with this view, recent studies on emotional behaviour and DS (see chapter 3) provide evidence to support the idea that at least for some people with DS, it is possible to identify a cognitive divergent affective processing style, as well as a cognitive divergent emotional meaning style (Morales and Lopez, 2006, 2010). From these considerations a larger question immediately emerges: *are they indeed emotionally different?*

Obviously, persons with DS are human beings like the rest of us, and because of this they are capable of experiencing the same spectrum of emotions we do. Every day, individuals with this syndrome, regardless their race, culture, age, etc., experience happiness, fear, anger, sadness, etc. In many circumstances, like other persons, they can use their common sense to infer the nature of their emotions (e.g., pleasant or unpleasant). However, for most of them, it is not always an easy task to identify the nature of negative emotions and frequently they have difficulties regulating their negative emotionality in a functional way. The specific reasons for this difficulty remain unclear. In fact, the complete range of specific DS emotional traits remains undetermined. As we will be arguing next, the scientific exploration of DS emotional behaviour has deep implications to better understand our own emotional world. In doing so, a two-step procedure will follow. First, a review of the current relevant academic literature outlining our understanding of the human emotion nature will be introduced. This will empower us to consistently frame and discuss seminal observations about a possible DS emotional phenotype.

2.2. The Emotional Nature of Human Beings: Basic Concepts

Emotions have been an important part of our human condition since ancestral times. Every day, we see examples of how people experience emotions and how these impact their life. If you read newspapers or watch news on TV, you will be able to find striking examples of how people live or die for emotional reasons; in some cases the reasons make no sense to us. No doubt, emotions guide our lives (e.g., people are willing to pay for emotional entertainment as movies, football games, listening to music, buying a dog), allow us to maintain our relationships (e.g., love, empathy, etc.). They regulate our behaviours helping us to adapt to our social context as functional members.

Many aspects of our society have been built so we are able to emotionalize. Seemingly, people are never free from the depths of our surrounding emotional world. For example, in the early 17th century in countries like England, melancholy was adopted as a cultural mood; many human expressions of art were influenced by this emotional state. Certainly, the music and painting of this period were characterized by a dark mood. Later, in the 18th century this melancholic cult as portrayed by dolefulness and grief mood changed to a more optimistic view of a welcoming world (Stearns, 2008; Stets & Turner, 2008). So, in some sense, to reach a broader understanding of who we are and how do we find significance our world it is necessary to have a better understanding about our own emotional nature. Being conscious of the fact that we are emotional beings, empower us to understand each other. However, understanding what makes us emotional beings as we are is not an easy task.

At present, behavioural sciences are aware of the relevance of emotion to human life. This has resulted in an increased interest in exploring a wide spectrum of emotion properties (e.g., emotional behaviour and regulation: Gyurak, Goodkind, Kramer, Miller, & Levenson, 2012; Eder, 2011; emotion cognitive mechanisms: Lichtenstein-Vidne, Henik, & Safadi, 2012; expression: Shariff & Tracy, 2011; Roch-Levecq, 2006; perception: Curby, Johnson, &

Tyson, 2012; Toffolo, Smeets, & van den Hout, 2012) throughout different perspectives (quantitative vs. qualitative), methods and instruments (e.g., see experimental designs: Lench, Flores, & Bench, 2011; surveys: Begeer, Banerjee, Rieffe, Terwogt, Potharst, Stegge & Koot, 2011; natural observations: Slatcher & Trentacosta, 2011, etc.) diversity of samples (e.g., see with typical conditions: Ponari, Conson, D'Amico, Grossi, & Trojano, 2012; Poirel, Cassotti, Beaucousin, Pineau, & Houdé, 2012; emotional disorders: Gruber, Oveis, Keltner, & Johnson, 2011; mental disorders: Wuerker, 1996; sensorial disabilities: Roch-Levecq, 2006, etc.) across several countries (e.g., see Elfenbein, Mandal, Ambady, Harizuka & Kumar, 2002). This research portrait visualizes humans as being provided with universal as well as individual biological and psychological mechanisms underlying their emotional nature. If something can be derived from this intense research activity, it is the necessity to expand our understanding about human emotion. For example, more information is needed regarding how this system varies when there are atypical neural, developmental or cognitive conditions.

At the center of this concern for more research on atypical emotion development are the people with DS themselves. They seem to have a divergent emotional awareness, and their sense of belonging and conception of the world appears to take a different emotional overtone from that of typical emotional views. Everyday observations emphasizing this emotional behaviour are frequently reported by parents, relatives and teachers, who work every day with members of this population. Nevertheless, determining to what extent this is truth represents a challenging enterprise to scientists studying human emotion, for at least two reasons. One reason is related to the progress of current scientific study of emotion, and another reason regards the methodological difficulties in studying DS emotion. Let us introduce some selected theoretical considerations related to these two concerns.

2.2.1. What is Emotion?

Not a long time ago, emotion was not considered relevant to the study of human nature; it was considered only a residual vestige from our evolutionary past (Morales et al., 2010). Nowadays scientific scrutiny has reallocated the study of emotion to the center of heated psychology academic debates that, among other things, consider the definition, nature, components and dimensions of emotion (e.g., see discussion on emotion by Widen & Russell, 2010; Izard, 2010; Izard, 2007).

The renewed interest on the topic of emotion in the last few centuries, complemented by the progress on neuroscience and the development of new research technology, have contributed to the creation of a wide range of definitions for emotion (Table 2.1). Plutchik (2001) estimated that through the 20th century, more than 90 emotion definitions were generated. In fact, Kleinginna and Kleinginna (1981) specified 92 definitions and 9 skeptical statements for the term of emotion. In general, they observed at least eleven different kinds of definitions based on: 1) the experiential categories of affect 2) the cognition, 3) physical categories of external emotional stimuli, 4) physiological mechanisms, 5) emotional expressive behaviour, 5) disruptive effects, 6) adaptive effects 6) the multiaspect nature of emotional phenomena, 7) those that distinguish emotion from other processes, 8) those that emphasize the overlap between emotion and motivation and 11) skeptical or disparaging statements about the usefulness of the concept of emotion.

Table 2.1. A list of emotion definitions to briefly illustrate the wide range of concepts used to define emotion (e.g., feelings, mechanisms, action patterns, process, functions), and the changing course of the emotion vision across the time

Author	Emotion's definitions
James (1884, *p. 190*)	He proposed that "*The bodily changes follow directly the perception of the exciting fact, and that our feeling of the same changes as they occur is the emotion*".
Watson (1916, *p. 596*)	He commented: "*To me an emotion is a bodily state which can be observed in man and animal equally well, such as the bristling of hair, shedding of tears, increase or decrease in respiration, sighing, heightened muscular activity, and the like. Some day we shall be able to mark off these objective states and classify them with respect to the types of stimuli which call them out (sex, food, shelter, noxious odors, etc*
Schachter and Singer (1962, *p. 380*)	They suggested that "*an emotional state may be considered a function of a state of physiological arousal and of a cognition appropriate to this state of arousal*".
Ortony, Clore & Collins (1988, *p.13*)	They considered emotions to be "*valenced reactions to events, agents, or objects, with their particular nature being determined by the way in which the eliciting situation is construed*".
Plutchik (2001, *p. 345-346*)	He wrote "*an emotion is not simply a feeling state. Emotion is a complex chain of loosely connected events that begins with a stimulus and includes feelings, psychological changes, impulses to action and specific, goal-directed behaviour. That is to say, feelings do not happen in isolation. They are responses to significant situations in an individual's life, and often they motivate actions*".
Oatley (2004, *p. 3*)	She argued that "*emotions are most typically caused by evaluations – psychologists also call them appraisals – of events in relation to what is important to us: our goals, our concerns, our aspirations*".

Although the question posed nearly 130 years ago by Willam James (1884) about what is an emotion remains open, scientific research efforts have made remarkable theoretical advances in understanding the structure, function and dynamic of human emotions. This kind of progress, framed by intense disagreements to how to conceptualize a study object like emotion, is not new to psychology. Take for instance the case of human intelligence. Psychologists have elaborated sophisticated models of human intelligence, despite not having a complete agreement about what intelligence is.

With regard to the scientific exploration of the DS emotional system, this has been generally carried on as individual/separate efforts without anyone considering an integrative approach. Fortunately, we should not to worry too much, since new multidisciplinary research efforts are prone to integrate previous research efforts. This is the case for integrative views of emotional development and DS (e.g., Sroufe, 1998) as well as the study of emotional neural structures related to the syndrome (e.g., electroencephalogram: Conrad, Schmidt, Niccols, Polak, Riniolo, & Burack, 2007; Magnetoencephalograph: Virji-Babul, Moiseev,

Cheung, Cheyne, Ribary, & Weeks, 2012, computer simulations, Morales & Lopez, 2012, etc.). Furthermore, advances in the conceptualization of emotion are framed by a renewed interest in exploring automatic appraisal mechanisms of emotional components (e.g., automatic processing of emotion: Morales & Lopez, 2010). However, in order to properly deal with the breadth of the academic spectra on DS and emotion, it is necessary first to enclose it using some theoretical developments on emotion theory that are sufficient to frame a DS emotional phenotype.

2.2.2. Some Emotion Theory

Current academic research on emotion is typified by a variety of theories, some of which are listed in Table 2.2. The list is not an exhaustive account of all of the theories on emotion, but it does serve our initial purpose of exploring the DS emotional world.

Consider from the previous table that there is no such thing as a single theory of emotion, but rather, the concept of emotion has been approached and explained using a variety of theoretical perspectives. Because of this, problems and limitations to one theory were frequently inherited in conceptualizion of emotion (Power & Dalgleish, 2008). Current emotion theory demands acknowledgement of these vestiges of theoretical and methodological limitations that are no longer a part of its current explanatory power. Considering the scientific study of atypical emotion development such as in DS to date, it is clear there are new possibilities in understanding emotion not only in this population but in all humans. This theoretical development can be achieved if previous bias to view atypical development just like a simple abnormality is reconsidered as an alternative biologically constrained mind-route to psychologically signify emotional worlds. As will be argued next and in the following chapters, cognitive methodology can be introduced and expanded to this inclusive theoretical intent which is a distinctive characteristic throughout this book, with a focus in Chapter 3.

2.2.3. Is There a Taxonomy for Emotions?

Every day, throughout the day, people have to deal with their own emotional experiences. Sometimes you may hear your friends or relatives verbally describing these experiences with, "I am very happy for you" or "I am angry at you", or with more global descriptions as "I feel very bad", or "I do not know". Most people effortlessly identify the nature of their emotion. For them, categorizing emotions (e.g., happiness, sadness, etc.), is not a big deal. However, there are persons among us who have difficulty recognizing and identifying their own emotional experiences (see discussion in Barrett, 2006). Emotion scientists seem to belong to this last group since the history of the scientific analysis of human emotion is plagued by heated debates regarding whether emotions can be organized into clearly distinguishable psychological categories (e.g., see proposals from Ekman, 1972; Izard, 1971) or if emotion should be defined as a continuum with dimensions (e.g., see Russell, 2003; Watson & Tellegen, 1985). Fortunately, both approaches (categorical and dimensional) have generated a wide range of research work to support their postulates, and as different they may appear, they frequently have common concerns, one of which is to elucidate whether or not there are kinds of emotion.

Table 2.2. Some theoretical approaches to the study of human emotion (adapted from Morales, 2010)

Theoretical approachs	Generalities	Examples
Early theories	First approaches to study emotion considered social and biological factors to distinguish it from non-emotional behaviour. Moreover, evolutive, physiological and functional aspects of emotion are a main focus (Strongman, 2003).	• McDougall's theory • James-Lange's theory • Cannon-Bard's theory • Papez's theory
Behavioural theories	Subjective components of emotions are not considered. Only behavioural components of emotion directly observable and measurable over time used as potential definitions to emotions. (English, 1924; Strongman, 2003).	• Watson's theory • Harlow-Stagner's theory • Millenson's theory
Developmental theories	Overall, a developmental perspective of emotion implies understanding the way of how emotional behaviour is organized through a time line (Srofue, 1998; Strongman, 2003).	• Socio-emotional theory of Sroufe • Giblin's Equilibrium theory of emotional development • Attachment theory of Bowlby
Social theories	Here, the emotion ethology is enclosed in social interaction contexts (e.g. social relationships, group expressions, etc.; see Strongman, 2003).	• The dictionary theory by Davitz • Social relationships theory by Rivera • Theory of dimensionality by Frijda • Weiner's attributional theory of emotion
Cognitive theories	Emotion is explained by internal psychological processes and the functional relation of these processes to social and context-adaptive demands. In doing so, specificity of emotion appraisal processes or mental representations of emotion schemata may be considered relevant cognitive components to emotion (e.g., Dalgleish & Power, 2000; Eich, Kihlstrom, Bower, Forgas & Niedenthal, 2000)	• Bower's network theory • Emotional appraisal theories
Cognitive science theories	Different explanatory levels converge to explain emotion. Neurocomputational, artificial intelligence, physics, neuroscience, linguistics and other scientific disciplines are systematically considered to provide research guidelines to study emotion (Bly & Rumelhart, 1999).	• Connectionist theory

Table 2.3. Examples of emotion taxonomies

Axis classification	Classification	Authors
	Emotions are focused on events, agents, or objects.	Ortony, Clore & Collins (1988)
Developmental status	Physiologic prototype/ precursory emotion/ Fundamental emotions/ maturing emotions	Sroufe (1998)
Dimensional	Positive/negative High/ low	Russell (1980)
Dimensional	Joy/Sadness Acceptance/Disgust Anger/Fear Surprise/Anticipation	Plutchik (1994)
	Pleasantness/Unpleasantness	Wilhelm Wundt (1896)
Dimensional	Strain / Relaxation Arousing / Subduing	
	Primary/secondary/ tertiary	Parrot (2001)
Categorical	Basic emotion	Ekman (1994)
	Basic emotion episodes/ emotion schemas	Izard (2009)

Classifying our emotions is a major challenge since they are not physical objects with properties easy to measure. As a matter of fact, there are still unresolved issues to identify what exactly they are. In addition, in order to establish a comprehensive and clear classification of emotion, it should be considered that emotion types could comprehend a variety of forms where the word emotion is referring to a group or family no just one of them (Ortony et al., 1988). As a result of this complexity and the differences among theoretical approaches a considerable number of emotional categorizations (see Table 2.3.) is obtained.

Here, our current goal is to frame DS emotions as a primary interest encompassing the "*basic emotions family*" (bottom of the table). This emotional set is proposed as the necessary and sufficient brain-mind-emotion system where any emotional system develops (human/nonhuman). According to Izard (2007b p.261-262), basic emotions are a group of neural, bodily/expressive, and feeling/motivational components that are produced automatically and nonconsciously as the result of evolutionarily adapted neurobiological and mental processes, activated by interaction between an affective–cognitive process and the sensing or perception of an ecological stimulus.

Inside a general functional consensus, basic emotions are assumed to be evolutionary old and essential for adaptation. In accordance with this view, there is compelling evidence supporting the idea of inherited emotion capacities. For instance, inherited primary emotion processing circuits for fear or anger activation that do not report their activity directly to higher regions of the brain can be identified (Pankseep, 1998, 2007). These emotion circuits can be triggered automatically and nonconciously. Supporting evidence to this concept are children without a cerebral cortex (Merker, 2007) capable of expressing and recognizing emotion and elemental primary emotion consciousness. Also, congenitally blind children are capable of emotion expression (Roch-Levecq, 2006). In other words, developmental context or cultural factors do not modify these subcortical emotion processing systems. Rather, basic emotions seem to be the building blocks of a subsequent sophisticated emotional system in maturity (from a constructivist view). Due to its evolutionary relevance and to the fact that these emotions are biologically constrained (Izard, 2007a) they are also typified as natural kinds (Izard, 2007b).

Although, the empirical data corpus obtained from different study approaches (e.g., cross-cultural studies of the facial expression of emotion, studies of the sequence of development of emotions, linguistic analyses of emotion terms, from categorization studies of emotion terms, from psychophysiological recording, studies of brain imaging) suggest the existence of basic emotions (Power & Dalgleish, 2008), there is still a strong criticism to this concept (Ortony, A., & Turner, 1990; Fridlund, 1997; Barret, 2005; Barrett, Lindquist, Bliss-Moreau, Duncan, Gendron, Mize & Brennan, 2007). Furthermore, even among the supporters of basic emotions idea there is not a completely agreement about how many basic emotions exist. It has generated a wide range of others list about basic emotions (e.g., see Ortony & Turner, 1990). For example, Dr. Paul Ekman in his seminal research (1992a, 1992b, 1992c) proposed that just a small set (see Table 2.4.) of emotions could be considered as basic and universal in humans (Ekman, 1994b, 1999). It is important to bear in mind that although not everyone agrees with this list (e.g. Sabini & Silver, 2005), there is extensive cross-cultural research supporting it.

Table 2.4. Ekman's basic emotions proposal

Basic emotions		
Original list	**Modified list**	
Anger	Contempt	Relief
Disgust	Shame	Satisfaction
Fear (awe)	Guilt	Sensory pleasure
Sadness/distress	Embarrassment	Contentment
Surprise	Amusement	
Enjoyment	Excitement	
	Pride in achievement	

Accordingly, to categorize an emotion as "basic", authors like Ekman and others (e.g., see Ekman, 1994b, 1999) proposed taking into account specific criteria for inclusion. In particular, Ekman (1994b, 1999) suggests the following list (Table 2.5.).

Table 2.5. Ekman's criteria for basic emotions

Criterions for basic emotions	
Specific characteristics	**General qualities**
Distinctive universal signals	Quick onset
Distinctive physiology	Brief duration
Distinctive subjective experience	Unbidden occurrence
Distinctive universals in antecedent events	Automatic appraisal, tuned to:
Distinctive appearance developmentally	Presence in other primates
Distinctive thoughts, memories images	

We would gladly discuss each of Ekman's criteria in depth, and certainly one single chapter alone would not be enough to explain the implications of each delimitation criterion. Nevertheless, we will intentionally focus on one single criterion relevant to our current chapter goal: the "distinctive universal signals" criterion that implies information processing constrains such as "rapid onset" and "automatic appraisal". For instance, one distinctive universal signal could be the facial display connected with a basic emotion (Izard, 1992, 1994; Ekman, Friesen, O'Sullivan, Chan, Diacoyanni-Tarlatzis, Heider, Krause, LeCompte, Pitcairn, Ricci-Bitti, Scherer, Tomita & Tzavaras, 1987; Ekman & Rosenberg, 2005). Among the most common expressions categorized as basic facial emotions are happiness, sadness, anger, disgust, fear and surprise (Figure 2.1.).

Ekman has provided empirical evidence for the universal character of these emotions throughout cultures and the different stages of human development. Regarding this categorical property of emotion, basic emotions have been explored inside the population with DS more than any other emotional aspect. Although, it should be noticed that the number of researches within the DS field is modest if is compared with those researchers in other of populations. Interestingly, the available evidence suggest that people with DS seems to have difficulties recognizing negative emotional faces as angry and surprise, which are supposed to be basic and universal.

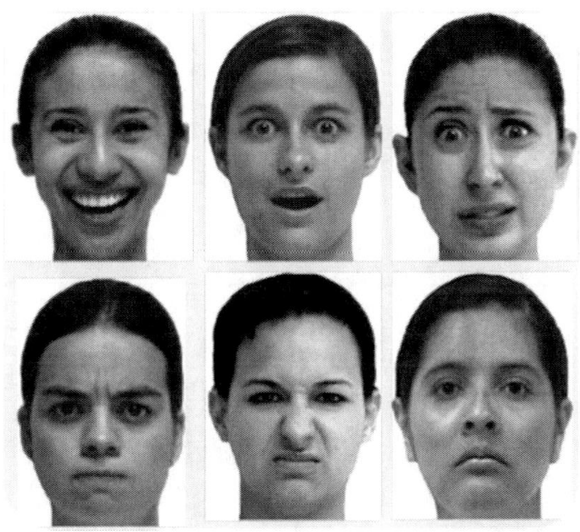

Figure 2.1. Young people from a typical population displaying instances of the basic emotion spectrum.

Interesting inquiries guiding exploration on the DS emotional nature are related to the underlying emotional structure in this population. Regarding this, take note first that typical individuals when tested in emotional experience studies, they are not only capable to report discrete emotions but they can organize them into a specific dimensional spherical emotional structure known as the emotion circumplex (Russell, 1980) (Figure 2.2. provides an example).

This well-documented pattern of emotional organization supports a dimensional model of affect in which the affective state of a person tends to be organized in a bi-dimensional space using two basic axes (see Figure 2.3.). The vertical axis is related to emotion valence (a pleasure–displeasure continuum) and the horizontal axis represents the dimension of arousal or alertness.

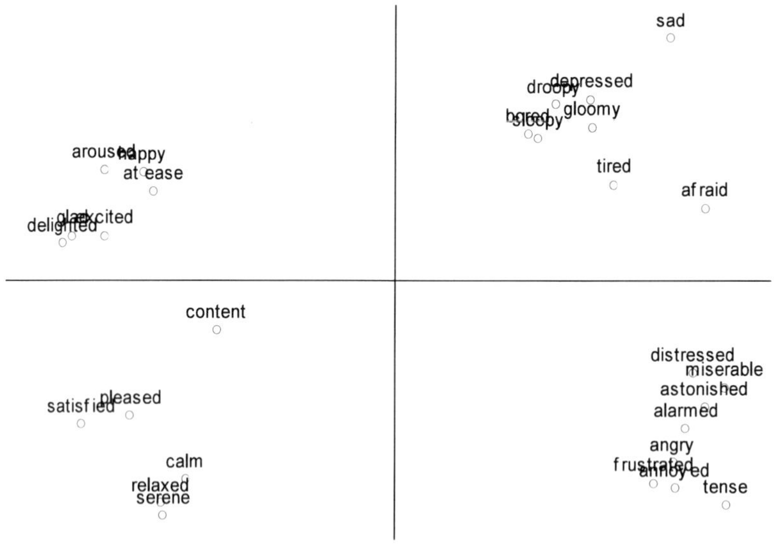

Figure 2.2. Emotional organization of an adolescent Mexican woman on two dimensions: pleasure-displeasure (horizontal axis) and degree of arousal (vertical axis).

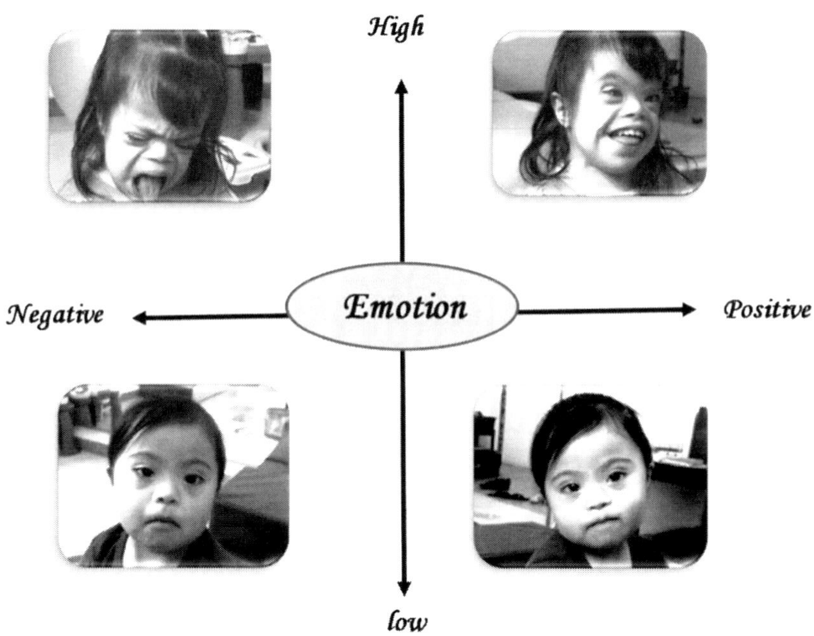

Figure 2.3. Human emotion dimensions organized in a bi-dimensional space. Vertical axes comprehend the emotional arousal or intensity and the horizontal axes refer to the emotional polarity or valence.

A considerable number of studies were carried out to prove this dimensional model on children, adolescents and adults from typical population. However, almost no research interest is found whenever atypical emotion development is considered, like in DS. This area seems to remain unexplored. Apparently, only Morales and Lopez (2012) have collected initial evidence on this topic on DS through facial emotional categorization tasks using the emotion circumplex mapping technique (see Russell, 1980, 1986). Their results suggest that some people with DS present the same circumplex emotional organization as those from the typical development population. However, some people with DS seem to differ from typical ones (See the emotional experience section in this chapter).

Additional research efforts from a cognitive point of view suggest some kind of divergent emotional processing of negative valence information in DS, specifically, a particular relation between levels of emotion arousal and appraisal mechanisms (Morales & Lopez, 2010; Morales, 2010; Morales & Lopez, 2006; Morales & Lopez 2004) (for more detail see next chapter). More discussion on this topic will be introduced later.

From the above it can be observed that both approaches can be useful in studying emotion and DS. For example, the dimensional approach to emotion has proven to be useful to account for a wide range of emotional phenomena (e.g., mood states: Watson & Tellegen, 1985; mood disorders: Gray 1982; Power & Dalgleish, 2008). Carrying on studies from a dimensional perspective can provide us not only with information about how people with DS organize their emotions, but allows us to obtain knowledge on mood states and disorders inside a DS condition. On the other hand, categorical views of human emotion are more suitable to explain cognitive processing like emotion learning. For instance, associative concept network theories (including emotion concept nodes) are capable of accounting for a wide variety of psychological phenomena related to codification and organization in memory as well as meaning construction (Murphy, 2002). Through this perspective, questions about how people with DS build emotional meaning could be explored.

Before describing possible applications of both views (categorical and dimensional) to study emotion in DS, a final concern regarding our own emotion nature will be discussed.

2.2.4. Emotional Components and Domains

No doubt, human emotion is a very complex phenomenon that is embraced by a very intricate physical system, which involves a wide variety of elements (e.g., physiological disturbance, changes in facial expression, gestures, behaviours, particular types of thoughts, beliefs, and desires, and a range of other experiences). Thus, our discussion will take the view that human emotion comprehends different components (biologic, cognitive, behavioural and contextual factors as the social environment), all of them taking part on the emotional domains of human life (emotional expression, experience, regulation, perception) (see Figure 2.4).

The denoted four domains in Figure 2.4 can be used to frame an emotional DS phenotype (e.g., how they experience and perceive the emotion). Facing this scientific challenge, it is recommendable to follow Plutchik's wise suggestion that "the place to start might be with the definition problem" (2001, p. 345).

The term "emotional phenotype" should be first defined. Here, the DS emotional phenotype is understood as the set of emotional behaviours, processes and traits that are specifically attributable to this genetic condition. Considering this initial conceptual we are ready now to introduce emotional aspects from the DS emotional world.

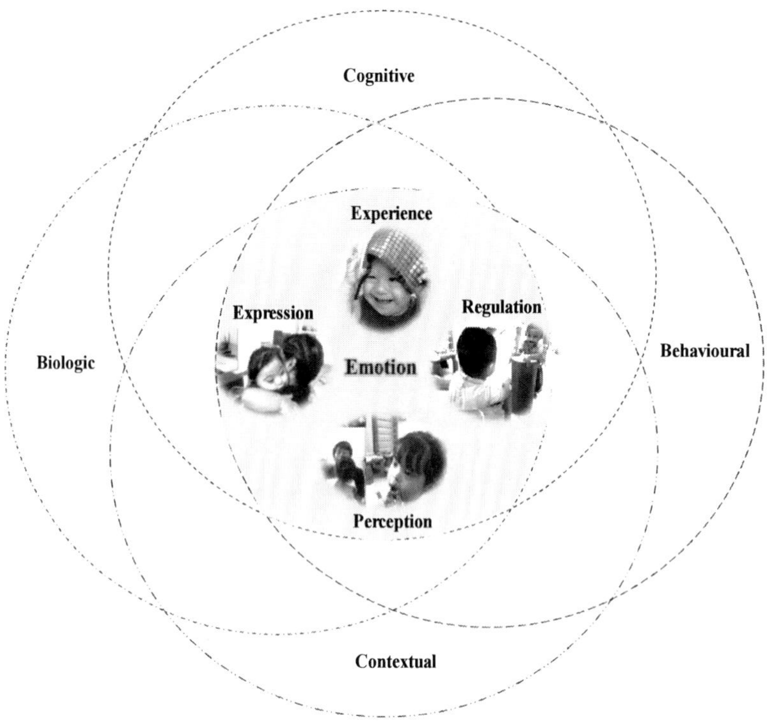

Figure 2.4. Emotion resulting from the intersection among different implicit and explicit domains of the human psychological life.

2.3. Generalities on the Down Syndrome Emotional Phenotype: Emotional Beings by Nature or Nurture

As it has been pointed before, studying the DS emotional system might lead to new ways of understanding the human emotional world. For example, it has been suggested that human intellectual disability (ID) is relevant to understanding the relationship between cognition and emotion (Sroufe, 1998). There are around 750 genetic conditions related to ID (Hodapp, DesJardin & Ricci, 2003), and DS is one of the biggest groups, almost one third of the entire ID population, and whose etiology is well known (Pitcairn & Wishart, 2000; Wishart & Pitcairn, 2000).

In particular it is well known that recruited DS neural architecture (frontal lobe, limbic temporal cortex, etc.) for information emotion processing has different anatomical and physiological characteristics from that of the typical population's neural circuitry (Jeringan, Bellugi & Sowell, 1993; Lubec, 2003; Raz, Torres & Briggs, 1995). This opens a door to unique scientific exploration to observe neurocognitive emotional functioning under atypical conditions. Even so, determining a DS emotional phenotype remains only a possibility. Scientific exploration to date has been concerned with DS semiology (Pace, Lynm & Glass, 2001; Pennington, Moon, Edgin, Stedron & Nade, 2003; Roizen & Patterson, 2003), its behavioural and cognitive implications (Cosgrave, McCarron & Anderson, 1998; Sroufe,

1998) as well as social consequences (Sroufe, 1998; Von Salisch, 2001). Only recently has academic attention inside the field of psychology been brought to systematically explore DS emotional behaviour (Carvajal & Iglesias, 2000; Einfeld, Tonge, Turner, Parmenter & Smith, 1999; Reddy, Williams & Vaughan, 2001; Sroufe, 1998; Von Salisch, 2001). To understand this new interest on DS behaviour and its implications to emotion science and the determination of a DS emotional phenotype let's consider the following discoveries on DS emotional behaviour.

2.3.1. Emotional Expression in Persons with DS

Human beings are not only capable of feeling emotions, but also they can express their quality and intensity, and understand them in others. Thus, emotional expression entails relevant information about internal states that work as social signals (Campos & Mumme, 1994), and also they allow us to elicit emotions in us and others (Shariff & Tracy, 2011). This can be devised from the following interview fragment from a father that has girl with DS:

> "Twenty days ago, I received a request to give a talk regarding Down syndrome. I invited my daughter (a very young woman with DS) to attend this talk…at the end of my speech I asked the audience to listen to the poetry recited by my daughter. A very deep feeling of pride wrapped me when all of the audience stood up and applauded my daughter; they were astonished, as if her performance would have been one huge enterprise…"

This example is very illustrative of the power of emotional expression. The child with DS was capable to have an emotional effect on the audience through her emotionally stirring poetry. And the audience expressed back to her their admiration with very emotional applause.

Since Charles Darwin (1872) published his book "The Expression of Emotions in Man and Animals", there has been a passionate discussion about functions, span and universality of emotional expression. From this debate, some derived theoretical considerations to emotional expression are:

a) Regardless of genetic condition, the connection between expression and emotion is varied by modality (e.g., body, facial, vocal) (Ekman, 1999), quality and quantity dimensions (e.g., frequency, intensity, etc.).
b) Not all expressions are emotionally genuine; some of them are social signals.
c) The universal character of the relation between emotion and expression does not state to what aspect of emotion the expression is connected. For example, it could be what is perceived at the face, the experienced feelings, the physiological changes, the memories and plans, or the particular social context (Ekman, 1999).

DS represents a very important area to explore in cognition and emotion under atypical development conditions. Studies in this area are scarce and have been mainly focused on facial expression (e.g., see Reddy, Williams & Vaughan, 2002; Smith & Dodson, 1996, Thompson, Cicchetti, Lamb & Malkin, 1985). This is because DS facial expression is considered important to emotional development and socialization (Morales, Lopez & Hedlefs,

2010). Generally speaking, two very complex neural systems in the human brain have evolved to control facial muscles. One of them controls reflexive behaviour (e.g. jaw movement by the masseter and the temporalis muscles) related to consumatory behaviour, attack and defense. Here, symmetric face display is involuntary activated. Neural circuitry related to this facial behaviour (Fridlund, 1994; Lundquvist & Öhman, 2005) originates from deep in the cerebral striatum and have no direct connection to neocortex processing. On the other hand, voluntarily-controlled facial muscles are innervated by the face area of the motor cortex. This neural circuitry relates to fine-tuned muscle control around the mouth, and sound articulation can be assimilated into learned social behaviour to achieve personal goals (e.g. deception; Ekman & O'Sullivan, 1991; Ekman & Rosenberg, 2005).

Very early in life, we display emotional facial expression and persons with DS are not exceptions (see Figure 2.5.).

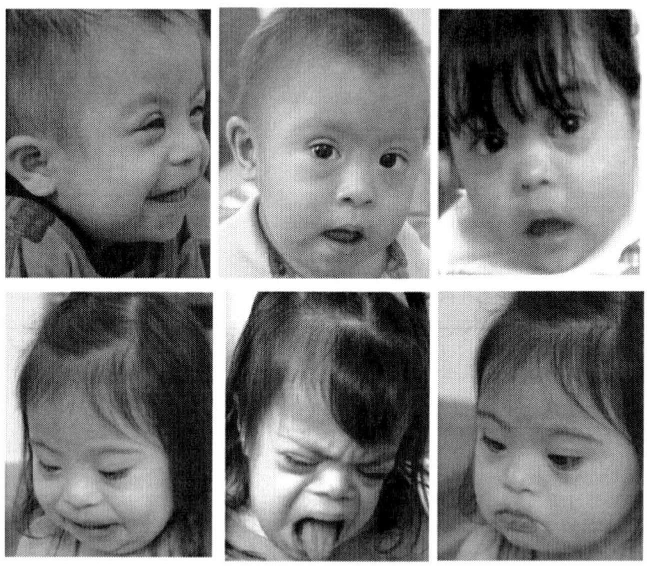

Figure 2.5. Children with DS between two and three years old show their capacity to display the basic emotion spectrum. Happiness, surprise and fear (top row). Disgust, anger and sadness (bottom row).

As can be deduced from Figure 2.5., children with DS can display basic emotional expressions (e.g., happiness, anger, sadness) with differing intensities and emotional valences. Although, some emotional developmental studies (Cicchetti & Beeghly, 1990; Cicchetti & Sroufe, 1976, 1978; Mans, Cicchetti & Sroufe, 1978) suggest that emotional expression strength and frequency seem diminished in children with DS compared with peers from the typical population. In particular, it has been observed that children with DS present a considerable development delay in social smiling. It tends to appear around 9 months and it seems to be expressed with less intensity and frequency compared to smile expression from typical development (TD) children. Interestingly, babies with DS' motives to laugh are chronologically arranged similarly as TD children. That is, first, they laugh due to intrusive auditory and tactile stimuli and only after these come laughter from more subtle social and visual stimuli.

Children with DS exhibit basic emotional expressions, and some of them seem to vary in properties of emotional expression such as intensity or frequency (e.g., smiling). However, emotion display and voluntary control of it are different aspects, and an immediate question emerges about voluntary emotional expression in this population. Persons with DS are frequently described as extraordinarily sincere persons, especially in the emotional aspect. Is this true, and if so, is this due to a regulation of emotion expression, constrained by their genetic condition?

It is useful to bear in mind when considering these questions, that early in life, emotional facial expressions are assumed to be involuntary and more genuine compared with those displayed in subsequent developmental stages. For babies, lying with facial expression does not bring as many benefits as sincere emotional expressions. However, humans need not only to be able to produce spontaneous facial expressions, but later on it becomes essential to produce voluntarily facial expressions as well.

However, facial expression is not only a genuine and direct channel to our internal emotional reality; it can be used in controlled ways as a device in social interactions. It is established that not all facial patterns occurring during interaction are truthful expressions of internal emotional states (Kaiser & Wehrle, 2001, Fridlund, 1997). For instance, people might become experts in deceiving others with their facial expressions, and sometimes it is hard to distinguish between genuine and deceptive emotion, especially if we do not have enough contextual information to do an accurate deception detection judgment (e.g. Castro, Lopez & Morales, 2012; Morales et al., 2010). Take as an example the faces in Figure 2.6.; try to recognize which facial expression is not genuine.

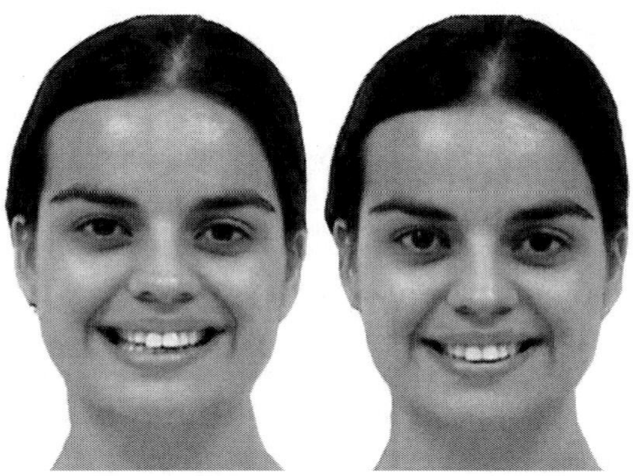

Figure 2.6. Examples of voluntary faking of (left panel) and genuine expression of a facial emotion (right panel).

Related to DS emotion expression, Morales and Lopez (2006, 2010, and 2011) have reported that whenever youngsters with DS are required to voluntarily smile, they have no difficulty doing so. However, expressing negative faces is different. In the study, a high percent of participants with DS failed to achieve the facial display. Only some participants managed to display negative facial expression (Figure 2.7).

The DS population shows variability about the ability to express emotion,which could be related to:

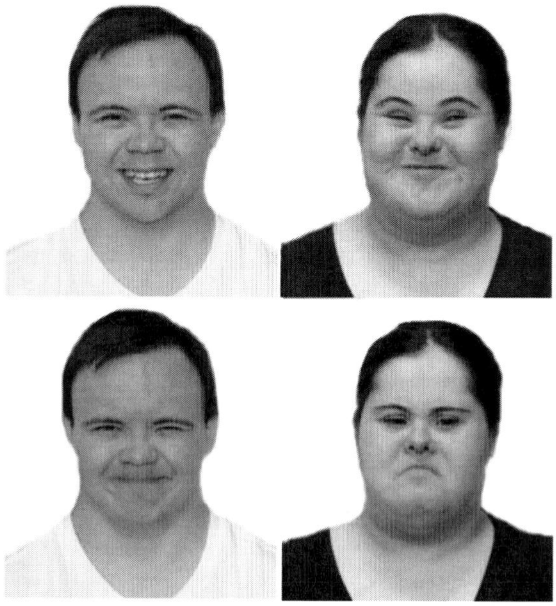

Figure 2.7. Youngsters with DS displaying a voluntarily smile in the top panel. One of these young adults had difficulty in voluntary displays of a negative face (e.g. angry) no matter how hard he tried (see left bottom panel), but the other youngster with DS was very capable of negative facial expression (see right bottom panel).

d) *Difficulties in negative emotion recognition.* Several authors have collected data suggesting that persons with DS posses a deficit in recognizing negative emotion. It is possible that some persons with DS cannot voluntarily produce a negative face (e.g., imitation tasks) due to their negative emotion recognition difficulties.

e) *Emotional style.* It has been suggested that persons with DS seem to prefer positive rather than negative information (Morales & Lopez, 2010). This preference could have an effect on their difficulty in producing negative expressions.

f) *The DS system to reproduce voluntarily* emotions *is not able* to do it accurately. For example, in Figure 2.7. The young man with DS perceives anger and he shows a very strong inclination to imitate this emotion however despite his efforts, almost a happy face prevails.

g) *Not full consciousness of their emotional expression.* It is possible that emotional self-monitoring processing is not working appropriately. In fact, in a study on familiar facial recognition of emotion, Morales and Lopez (2010) required participants with DS to produce negative expressions. If participants displayed a happy face instead of an angry expression they were shown their own face using a mirror, and were told that his/her emotional expression was not an angry expression. Some participants did not agree with this observation; they really believed they were displaying a negative emotion despite displaying what would be classified as a facial expression of happiness. However, the other participants recognized that their facial expression was not the required negative display.

The first three suggested explanations will be discussed in detail in Chapter 3. The final one has not been explored, but initial academic consideration could be influenced by it in considering modern theoretical background on emotion as is described later on.

2.3.2. Emotional Experience

Frequently, parents, teachers, friends and people who closely relate to persons with DS could be defined as a kind of experts to feel emotions since they seem to always experience emotions. Let us expand a little bit more on this aspect to show more of what we know about the emotional system of people with this genetic condition.

First, because persons with DS have the same emotional neurostructure as other human beings, there is no apparent reason why members of this population cannot feel the same range of human emotion. This can be exemplified by the following conversation fragments with a young adult with DS:

Conversation 1: Happiness

Interviewer: "How do you feel now?

Interviewee: I am very well, happy....

Interviewer: Why?

Interviewee: Happy because I work... my dad and mom are happy too...".

This young man finds great satisfaction working in a commercial center. He packs things people buy, and this is funny to him. He thinks it is very nice to work because his parents are happy for him too.

Conversation 2: Anger

Interviewer: Has anybody done something bad to you?

Interviewee: Of course, I am angry at [classmate name] now.

Interviewer: Why?

Interviewee: Because he ate some of my cookie... and after that, he ate the rest.

In this case a girl with DS expressing her anger because a classmate took her lunch.

Conversation 3: Worry/Fear

Interviewer: How are you?

Interviewee: Look... I am very worried, because... look, all people who I know are dying, I am afraid to die.... Why? I do not want that.

(**Interviewer** [big silence])

Here, an adult with DS expresses a profound concern about an inevitable life event.

These persons with DS were capable to experience emotions in simple or complex situations, but they were also perfectly capable of expressing the feelings they experienced. The ability to be aware of one's own emotional experiences is present in all members of this population. Moreover, it has been observed through several emotion studies from Morales and Lopez (2010, 2006) that even when some participants with DS have difficulties in defining what an emotion is, they can perfectly exemplify them. Interestingly, some of the considered sample participants with DS completely denied the possibility to feel anger (see Chapter 3). When these participants were requested to emulate or produce negative emotions some of them refused to do it. They argued that it wouldn't be possible since they are happy persons that never feel anger (as a curious thing some of these participants with DS expressed anger while denying the possibility of experiencing these kinds of emotion).

Now, how is it possible that they deny these negative emotions? The answer is not so simple. A person can be able to experience an emotion while not necessarily being able to perceive the emotion. In fact, some authors argue the existence of several levels of consciousness of emotional experience.

Regarding this, Izard (1977, 2007a, 2007b, 2009) suggests that emotions include a feeling component, that is, sensation of experienced neurobiological activity related to an emotion (see also Panksepp, 2005). Different levels of awareness of feeling are possible and thus an emotion feeling has different accessibility levels to consciousness. Thus, through basic emotions from the earliest stages of ontogeny, infants become aware of emotions, long before the appearance of self-conception and language conceptualization (Izard, Fantauzzo, Castle, Haynes, Rayias, Putnam, 1995). By dynamically linking basic emotions and basic emotion feelings to images and concepts young infants can form rudimentary *emotion schemas*. Later on, these memory structures will be responsible for associating words associated with labeling emotions and through the acquisition of language, reflexive behaviour, thinking and cultural influence, these emotion schemata become sophisticated.

These mature complex emotion schemas are the ones that an adult recognizes as emotions and not the basic emotions described earlier (see Figure 2.8.). Thus, basic negative emotions of anger or fear are initial emotional patterns that are the foundation for the emotion schemas to build more sophisticated angry or fearful emotions. More interestingly, basic emotion feelings are through emotion schemas that are direct precursors to our consciousness formation (Izard, 2007a, 2007b). Consequently, emotions lead to conceptual processes and consciousness rather than being sources of their origin. The kind of cognitions integrated into emotion schemas may include high level appraisal mechanisms that differentiate concrete emotions (Power & Dalgleish, 2008), and develop organized thinking (Eisenberg & Spinrad, 2004).

Now, it remains a long road for scientific exploration to travel before we can determine how basic emotions and schemata emotion link our cognitions to produce emotional consciousness and language. No doubt, the Down syndrome condition is an excellent prism that reflects an emotional spectrum useful to systematic behaviour analysis. Specifically, it is expected that the formation of a constrained negative-positive system during early ontogeny reflects its influence in consciousness through atypical behaviour. Take for instance, the case of blaming someone. This psychological activity requires the identification of negative behaviour. Since persons with DS seem to have difficulties recognizing negative information, it can be hypothesized that certainly social rules related to this blaming behaviour must be peculiar due to a different way of perceiving negativity. Insightful explorations contrasting DS blame processing versus typical blaming behaviour can be obtained. Morales, Charles, Castro, Lopez & Mullet (2012) carried on a study on this topic, and found that a considerable number of the participants with DS were able to evaluate negative events and to express blaming or judgments similar to the general population (see Chapter 4). Then consideration of a person with DS as an "eternal child" because of he or she has are not capable of responsible behaviour must be reevaluated since not all members of this population have difficulties in evaluating and using negative information, at least in everyday events.

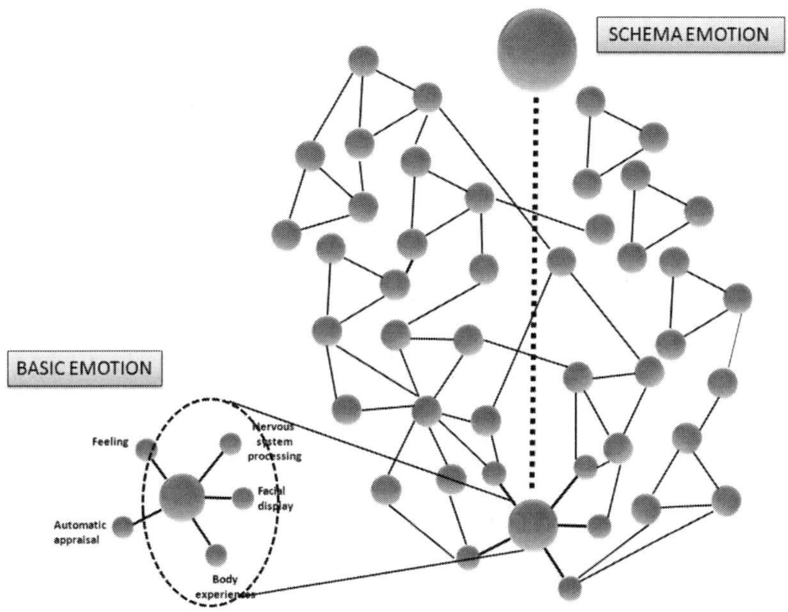

Figure 2.8. Schema emotions of anger, fear, etc., are built by dynamically linking basic emotions anger, fear, etc., to higher cognitive processing and linguistic process. It is due to this constructive cognitive-emotional processing that emotions are culturally differentiated and we acquire an emotional consciousness of our environment (e.g., Izard, 1977, 1992).

To all intents and purposes, the vision of a "deficit" in recognizing negative information is inappropriate as a research approach to explore DS emotional consciousness, since this vision could suggest, as the "sickness" vision suggested, that academic exploration must be oriented only to detect things supposedly to be wrong. Of course, under the deficit perspective, the DS emotional world seems not worth exploring. Consequently, systematic analysis of the emotional behaviour in this population demands us a more open-minded research approach. Some instances of new methodological views are illustrated in this book in the hopes that special education researchers might find insights they can then include in their own research either in DS or in other special education areas.

Moreover, by understanding the emotional world of persons with DS, their life opportunities can be expanded and developed. Specifically, their limited civil rights (e.g., marriage) could improve to new horizons. If you have had the opportunity to deal with members of this group you will immediately identify that the most important conversation topic (in teenagers and adults) is about being in love and getting married. Exhibiting romantic cheating behaviours or maintaining multiple romantic candidates before selecting a final romantic partner is not rare within members of this population. However, weighting the negative consequences of these behaviours seems to be different from that of a typical person (see Chapter 4).

The person with DS' emotional meaning construction represents a vast field to explore. Knowing how they signify emotional events will be a big advance in the nature's comprehension of their emotional experience. A first approach to this will be to determine how people with DS organize the emotional information in their memory. Memory science suggests that persons organize the information in conceptual networks — also known as semantic networks — since meaning about events or objects is built by spreading activation of semantic related concepts. These mental representations include pieces of emotional information too. For example, whenever we recognize someone who is familiar to us, we activate a set of semantically related concepts that may include emotional information, that is, discrete categorical emotion nodes (see Figure 2.9.).

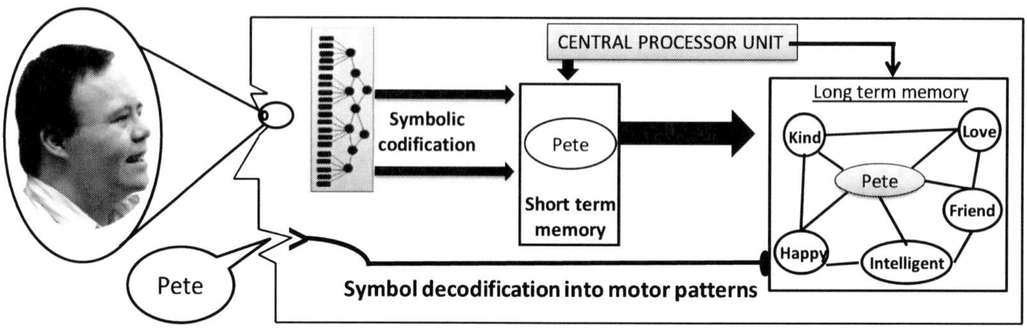

Figure 2.9. A display of a simplified Human Information Processing Model showing the semantic network activation (including emotion nodes) triggered by face recognition processing.

As it was proposed by Bower and colleagues (Bower & Forgas, 2000) emotional life events could be codified and organized in our memory by emotion nodes in a network and that at least 4 or 8 emotion nodes must be innately wired in our brains. These "basic" emotion nodes are biologically constrained and are triggered by relevant survival and adaptation environmental cues. These basic emotions are the conceptualization platform where the emotional world is built and culturally differentiated throughout an individual's lifespan (e.g. Fridlund, 1997; Keltner, Ekman, Gonzaga & Beer, 2003). Little is known about the construction and functioning of these emotion networks under the DS condition. However, it is assumed that a DS emotion network will serve the same purpose as that of a typical person, that is, emotional meaning construction to signify both the internal world as well as the outside world.

Gordon Bower's network theory of emotion (Bower, 1981, 1992; Bower & Cohen, 1982), proposes that the activation of one emotion node (e.g. happiness) might have inhibitory effects over another emotion node (e.g. Sadness) as it is described in Figure 2.10. It is postulated that the absence of such inhibitory effects in emotional networks could lead to emotional disorders.

Although Bower's theory presents several empirical and theoretical limitations (see Power & Dalgleish, 2008), it is a landmark for academic research to analyze attention, perceptual and memory bias processes related to emotion, and could be a very useful theory framework to begin to understand persons with DS' emotional world. For instance, consider emotion schemas where negative concepts do not inhibit or activate other concepts. It is expected that emotional network organization to have an effect not only on emotional meaning construction but over several controlled and automatic cognitive processes that are under schema-based control. Indirect evidence for this possibility can be obtained from affective priming studies (Morales & Lopez 2005, 2006, and 2010) that use categorization tasks where familiarity to faces affect automatic appraisal processing, specifically to positive stimuli (also, see the perception section in this chapter, and Chapter 3).

On the other hand, and as previously noted, dimensional approaches have proposed that emotion organization concepts can be analyzed through two-dimensional geometric representations based on two properties: valence (pleasure–displeasure) and arousal (activation–deactivation) (see Figure 2.3). There is evidence that these two dimensional properties organize the average person's emotional structure through a circular (or circumplex-type) shape (see Barrett, 2006; Barrett & Russell, 1999). This kind of pattern has been obtained with different kind of stimuli as words (see Figure 2.2) or facial expression (see Figure 2.8). As we mentioned before, at the present time no formal research can be found which considers dimensional DS emotion circumplex structure. Indeed there is little scientific exploration of emotional experience under atypical development conditions (e.g., intellectual disability: Geoffrey R. Argus, Peter C. Terry, Paul Bramston, Sarah L. Dinsdale, 2004).

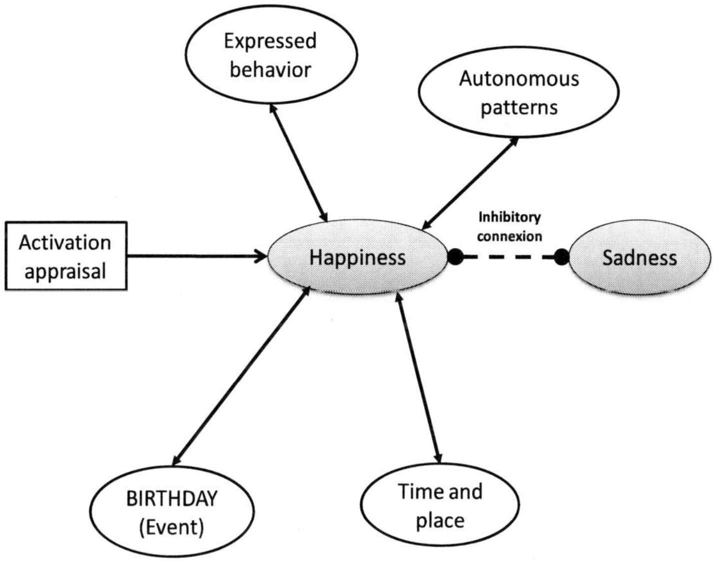

Figure 2.10. Controlled or automatic appraisal processing of a social event (a birthday party) is capable of emotion activation (happiness). Instant inhibition spreads to sadness. This mental representation is an emotion network model constrained by biological emotion nodes wired in our brain called basic emotions.

Recently, we carried out a pilot study on adults with DS' emotional structure based on the emotional categorization task by Russell and Bullock (1986). Participants were required to classify emotional faces into two, three and five groups based on similarity in emotional stimuli. First, as in the study of Russell and Bullock, ten different facial expression of emotion were selected (happiness, surprise, fear, anger, disgust, and sadness, excitement, calm, sleepiness, and boredom). In contrast to the original study, all facial expressions belonged to only one man (see Figure 2.9.). The reason for using just one person was because participants with DS had some difficulties in understanding the task if the emotional facial expressions were displayed by different persons. They grouped the faces by physical features and not for emotional similarity (no matter how much practice they had) or they refused to do the task since they considered that the important thing was to group people by physical attributes like being beautiful.

Photos of the ten emotional expressions were selected from Be-face (a free of charge emotion facial base, http://www.cognilab.org/RECURSOS.html; Morales & Lopez, 2010). The ten emotional expressions were randomly presented on a table and after the participant pointed at one, it was placed on table in front of she/he. Subsequently, the participant was required to select another face that was completely different to that one that she/he had previously chosen (see Figure 2.11.). This process was repeated, but now the participant was required to choose the three most different emotional faces.

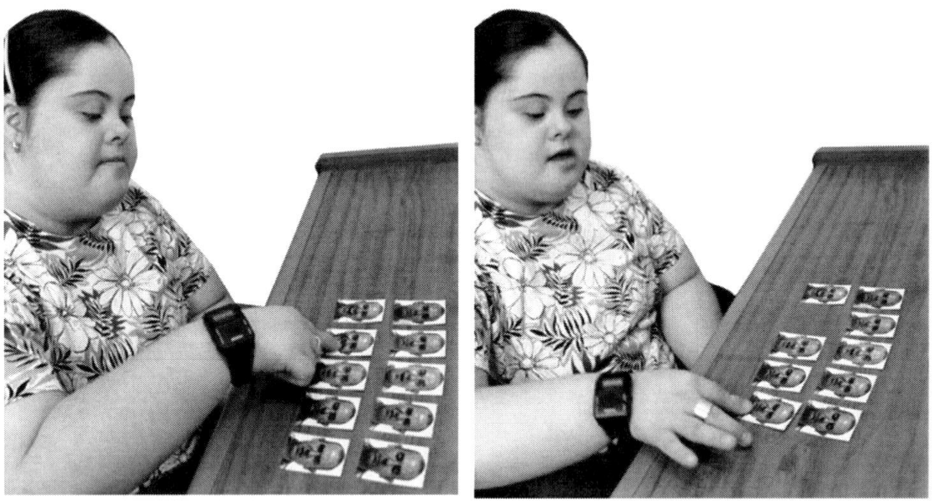

Figure 2.11. First phase example: selecting two emotional faces that are completely different. Participant selected a happy face then had to choose an expression not similar to happiness, such as anger.

In the second phase, the participant classified in two groups the ten faces according to similarity. In order to this, the experimenter placed the first two photos selected from the initial phase on the table in front of the participant. Then the experimenter randomly picked one photo from the eight remained and showed it to the participant. Here, she/he was required to look at the face and indicate if the person in the photo looked more like the person in the first photo or the second one (Figure 2.12.). The procedure for the third phase was similar. The three faces chosen by the participant in the first phase were placed in front of the person, and she/he classified the remained photos into three groups by similarity to these facial displays.

In the final phase, the participant categorized the faces in five groups based on similarity. Here, the researcher asked the participant to pick one face, which was then placed in front of the person. Then, she/he had to choose the face that expressed the more similar feeling. This procedure was repeated until five facial pairs were formed. As in the original Russell and Bullock's experiment, a similarity matrix was obtained from the scores of the three categorization phases. Figure 2.13. shows multidimensional scaling analysis examples of emotional organization of DS and typical persons (TD). In both DS cases, participants had good verbal skills and they presented mild intellectual disability. Note that only one person with DS could organize emotions according to Russell's predictions (like the TD participants' circumplex). Reasons for this variability are unexplored.

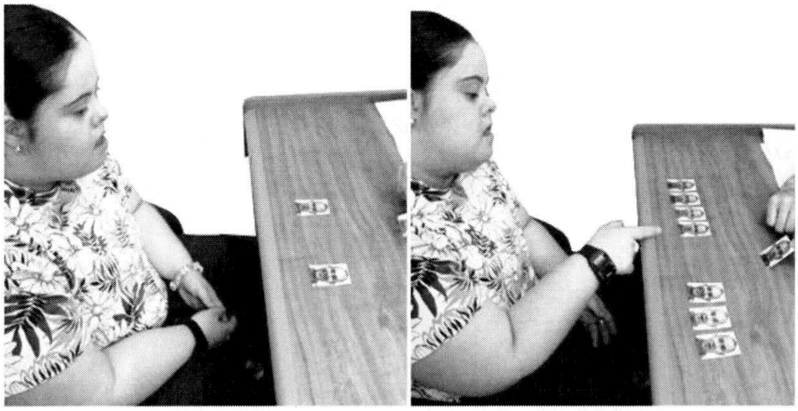

Figure 2.12. Second phase example: classifying emotional expressions into two groups.

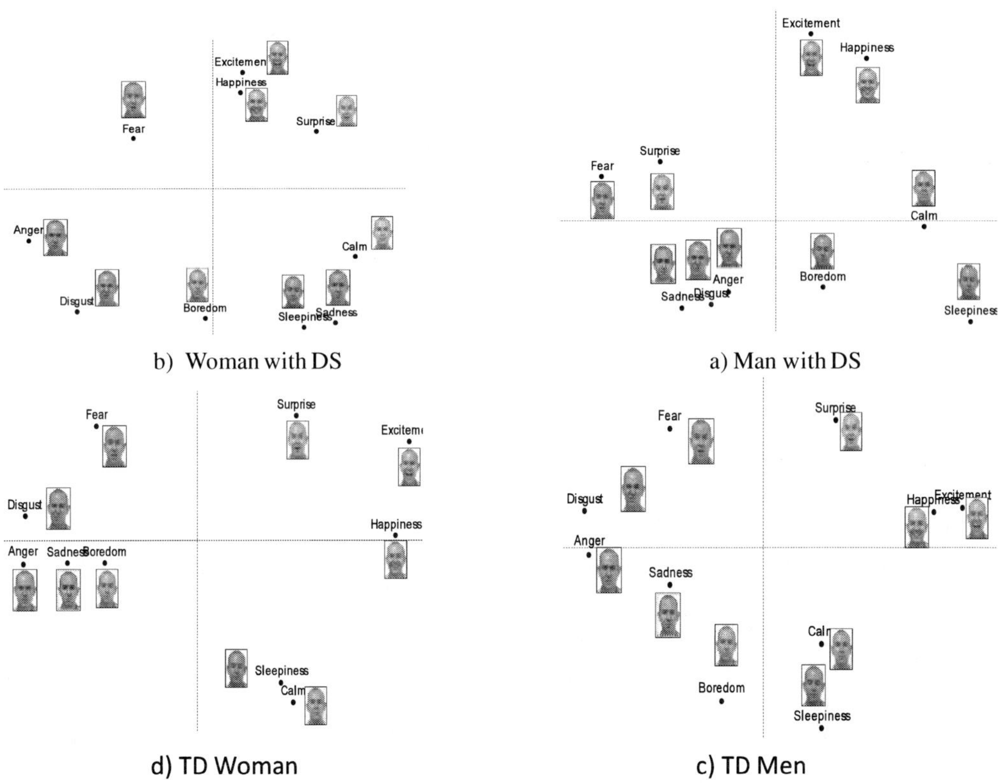

Figure 2.13. Emotional circumplex for four adult participants with DS and with typical development (TD) using emotional facial expression.

Altogether, evidence suggests that persons with DS can experience positive and negative emotions. Some of them may deny experiencing negative emotionality. Even thus they can organize most part of this kind of emotions as different from positive emotional experiences (not necessarily as opposite valence emotions as they are reviewed in the next chapter). On the other hand, some negative experiences as sadness seem to be classified as positive by some persons with DS (Figure 2.13.). This is interesting because as we will discuss later, affective priming research shows that some participants with DS that showed difficulties in recognizing negative expressions (e.g., anger, fear) could perfectly identify the sadness facial expression. Although the meaning of these observations remains unclear, we could say that this particular way of experiencing emotions typify DS emotional behaviour (see also emotional regulation, next). In fact, some authors have suggested that the way in which persons with DS experience emotions relates to their emotional expression and regulation (Smith & Walden, 1998). More academic research in this direction is needed regardless the academic approach (whether categorical or dimensional point of view).

2.3.3. Emotional Regulation

Persons with DS are described as warm, gentle and cheerful individuals. They are often thought to be easygoing with a great ability to form positive relationships with almost everyone (e.g. see Mundy, Sigman, & Kasari, 1990; Rosner, Hodapp, Fidler, Sagun, & Dykens, 2004; Freeman & Kasari, 2002; Dykens & Kasari, 1997; Meyers & Pueschel, 1987). At the same time, in addition to this stereotype, some authors report that persons with DS tend to display inappropriate emotional behaviours that favor their social exclusion or discrimination. For example, when it comes to social interaction, it is common to find that they tend to approach too much close to the person, and apparently do not understand or recognize disapproval to this behaviour (e.g., negative faces). For most of us this kind of emotional expressions is assumed to be a violation of a conventional social rule (social distance). These difficulties in managing emotional expression from others is related to their emotion regulation and affects social functioning, peer acceptance (e.g., see Wranik, Barrett, & Salovey, 2007; Eisenberg, Hofer, & Vaughan, 2007; Shaver & Mikulincer, 2007; Calkins, Gill, Johnson, & Smith, 1999; Eisenberg, Fabes, Guthrie, & Reiser, 2002), and even physical illness (Sapolsky, 2007).

Emotion regulation entails changes over a person`s emotional dynamics (Thompson, 1990), or systematic variation over the different emotion properties (e.g., emotion latency, rise time, magnitude, duration, and offset of responses from the behavioural, experiential, or physiological domains) to maintain, diminish or intensify emotion to achieve personal goals (Gross, 2007).

Developmental studies on emotion regulation observe that even when children with DS display similar types of emotional reactions as typical children with the same mental age, they behave differently over modulation of duration and intensity of emotional responses (see Cicchetti & Sroufe 1976; Serafica & Cicchetti 1976; Thompson, Cicchetti, Lamb, Malkin, 1985; Kasari et al. 1990; Kasari & Sigman 1996).

Overall, children with DS seem to use a restricted range of strategies, at least in situations where they need to cope with frustration (Jahromi, Gulsrud & Kasari, 2008), cognitively challenging tasks (Kasari & Freeman, 2001; Pitcairn & Wishart, 1994), delay of gratification tasks (Cuskelly et al., 2003; Kopp et al., 1983), etc. Unfortunately, little is known about their emotional regulation strategies in other aspects of adolescence and adulthood.

2.4. Final Words

The association between a specific genetic condition and a particular form to react or to behave is not by all means a new idea (e.g. Enfield, Tonge, Parmenter & Smith, 1999). Here, we have explored different domains of the emotional system taking into account the DS condition. Some authors have observed specific emotional behaviour patterns typical of DS (e.g., they display low emotional reactivity to the world when compared to typical development children). However, there is not enough information to complete an integral view of a DS emotional phenotype throughout all developmental stages. Although it is highly encouraging to observe a growing interest in exploring the emotional domains of this genetic condition. This brings the possibility of obtaining a more accurate view of the DS emotional world.

References

Barrett, L. F. (2005). Feeling is perceiving: Core affect and conceptualization in the experience of emotion. In L. F. Barrett, P. M. Niedenthal, & P. Winkielman (Eds.), Emotions: Conscious and Unconscious (pp. 255-284). New York: Guilford.

Barrett, L. F., & Russell, J. A. (1999). Structure of current affect. *Current Directions in Psychological Science, 8,* 10–14.doi: 10.1111/1467-8721.00003

Barrett, L. F. (2006). Solving the emotion paradox: categorization and the experience of Emotion. *Personality and Social Psychology Review,* 10(1), 20–46.

Barrett, L. F., Lindquist, K. A., Bliss-Moreau, E., Duncan, S., Gendron, M., Mize, J., & Brennan, L. (2007). Of mice and men: Natural kinds of emotions in the mammalian brain? A response to Panksepp and Izard. *Perspectives on Psychological Science*, 2, 297–312.

Begeer, S., Banerjee, R., Rieffe, C., Terwogt, M. M., Potharst, E., Stegge, H. &Koot, H. M. (2011).The understanding and self-reported use of emotional display rules in children with autism spectrum disorders. *Cognition & Emotion, 25*(5), 947-956. doi: 10.1080/02699931.2010.516924.

Bly, B. M. & Rumelhart, D. E. (Eds.). (1999). Cognitive science (2a. ed.). San Diego, California, EE. UU.: Academic Press.

Bower, G. H. & Cohen, P. (1982)._Emotional influences on learning and cognition._In M.S. Clark & S.T. Fiske (Eds.), *Affect and Cognition* (pp.291-331). Hillsdale, NJ: Laurence Erlbaum Associates.

Bower, G. H. & Forgas, J. P. (2000). Affect, memory, and social cognition. En E. Eich, J. F. Kihlstrom, G. H. Bower, J. P. Forgas& P. M. Niedenthal (Eds.). *Cognition and emotion* (pp. 87-168). Nueva York, NY, EE. UU.: Oxford Press.

Bower, G. H. (1981). Mood and memory. *American Psychologist, 36*(2), 129-148. doi:10.1037/0003-066X.36.2.129

Bower, G. H. (1992). How might emotions affect learning? In S.-A. Christianson (Ed.), *Handbook of emotion and memory* (pp. 3-31). Hillsdale, NJ: Erlbaum.

Calkins, S. D., Gill, K. L., Johnson, M. C., & Smith, C. L. (1999). Emotional reactivity and emotional regulation strategies as predictors of social behaviour with peers during toddlerhood. *Social Development*, 8, 310–334. doi: 10.1111/1467-9507.00098

Campos, J. J. & Mumme, D. L. (1994). A FUNCTIONALIST PERSPECTIVE ON THE NATURE OF EMOTION. Monographs of the Society for Research in Child Development, 59: 284–303. doi: 10.1111/j.1540-5834.1994.tb01289.x

Carvajal, F. & Iglesias, J. (2000). Looking behaviour and smiling in Down syndrome infants. *Journal of Nonverbal Behaviour, 24*(3), 225-236. doi: 10.1023/A:1006693121491

Castro, C.C., Lopez, R. E. O. & Morales, M. G. E. (2012). Cognitive algebra to deception detection: Information Integration Theory contributions to study human deception detection's cognitive nature. *International Journal of Psychology Research*, *7*(5/6), 1-11. Available from https://www.novapublishers.com/catalog/advanced_search_result.php?keywords=Claudia+Castro%2C+Ernesto+Octavi&x=0&y=0

Darwin, C. R. (1872). The expression of the emotions in man and animals. London: John Murray.

Cicchetti, D. & Beeghly, M. (1990). An organizational approach to the study of Down syndrome: Contributions to an integrative theory of development. In D. Cicchetti & M. Beeghly (Eds.), *Children with Down syndrome: A developmental perspective* (pp. 29-62). New York: Cambridge University Press.

Cicchetti, D. & Sroufe, L. A. (1976). The emotional development of the infant with Down syndrome. In J. L. Poor (Ed.), *Aim: To fight low expectations of Down's syndrome children* (pp. 37-59). Forest Lake, MN: Forest Lake Printing, Inc.

Cicchetti, D. & Sroufe, L. A. (1978). An organizational view of affect: Illustration from the study of Down's syndrome infants. In M. Lewis & L. Rosenblum (Eds.), *The development of affect* (pp. 309-350). New York: Plenum Press.

Cicchetti, D. & Sroufe, L. A. (1976). The relationship between affective and cognitive development in Down's syndrome infants. *Child Development, 47,* 920-929.

Conrad, N. J., Schmidt, L. A., Niccols, A., Polak, C. P., Riniolo, T. C. & Burack, J. A. (2007). Frontal electroencephalogram asymmetry during affective processing in children with Down syndrome: a pilot study. *Journal of Intellectual Disability Research, 51*(12), 988-995. doi: 10.1111/j.1365-2788.2007.01010.x

Cosgrave, M., McCarron, M. & Anderson, M. (1998). Cognitive decline in Down syndrome: a validity/reliability stufy of the Test for severe impairment. *American Journal on Mental Retardation, 103*(2), 193-197. Available from http://www.aaiddjournals.org/doi/abs/10.1352/0895-8017%281998%29103%3C0193%3ACDIDSA%3E2.0.CO%3B2

Curby, K. M., Johnson, K. J. & Tyson, A. (2012). Face to face with emotion*Cognition & Emotion, 26*(1), 93-102. doi: 10.1080/02699931.2011.555752

Cuskelly, M., Zhang, A. & Hayes, A. (2003). A mental age matched comparison study of delay of gratification in children with Down syndrome. *International Journal of Disability, Development and Education, 50,* 239-251. doi: 10.1080/1034912032000120435

Dalgleish, T. & Power, M. (Eds.) (2000). *Handbook of cognition and emotion*. Nueva York, NY, EE.UU.: John Wiley & Sons.

Dykens, E. M. & Kasari, C. (1997). Maladaptive behaviour in children with Prader-Willi syndrome, Down syndrome and non- specific mental retardation. Am J Ment Retard 102, 228-37. doi: 10.1352/0895-8017(1997)102<0228:MBICWP>2.0.CO;2

Eder, A. B. (2011). Control of impulsive emotional behaviour through implementation intentions. *Cognition & Emotion, 25*(3), 478-489. doi: 10.1080/02699931.2010.527493.

Eich, E., Killstrom, J. F., Bower, G. H., Forgas, J. P. & Niedenthal, P. M. (Eds.). (2000). *Cognition and emotion.* Nueva York, NY, EE. UU.: Oxford Press.

Enfield, S., Tonge, B.,Turner, G., Parmenter, T. & Smith, A. (1999). Longitudinal course of behavioural and emotional problems of young persons with Prader-Willi, Fragile X, Williams and Down syndrome. *Journal of intellectual and Development Disability, 24* (4): 349-354. Retrieved from http://www.eric.ed.gov/ERICWebPortal/search/detailmini.jsp?_nfpb=true&_&ERICExtSearch_SearchValue_0=EJ603344&ERICExtSearch_SearchType_0=no&accno=EJ603344

Eisenberg, N. & Spinrad, T. L. (2004). Emotion-related regulation: Sharpening the definition. *Child Development, 75*, 334–339.

Eisenberg, N., Fabes, R. A., Guthrie, I. K. & Reiser, M. (2002). The role of emotionality and regulation in children's social competence and adjustment. In L. Pulkkinen& A. Caspi (Eds.), *Paths to successful development: Personality in the life course* (pp. 46–70). New York: Cambridge University Press.

Eisenberg, N. Hofer, C. & Vaughan, J. (2007). Effortful control and its socioemotional consequences In J. Gross (Ed.), *Handbook of emotion regulation* (pp. 287–306.). New York: Guilford.

Ekman, P. & O'Sullivan, M. (1991). Who can catch a liar? *American Psychologist, 46*, 913-920.Retrieved from http://psycnet.apa.org/index.cfm?fa=buy.optionToBuy&id=1992-05387-001

Ekman, P. & Rosenberg, E. L. (2005). *What the face reveals: Basic and applied spontaneous expression using the Facial Action Coding System (FACS).* (2nd ed.) New York: Oxford University Press.

Ekman, P. (1972). *Emotions in the human face.* New York: Pergamon Press.

Ekman, P. (1992a). Are there basic emotions? *American Psychologist, 46*, 913-920. doi: 10.1037/0033-295X.99.3.550

Ekman, P. (1992b). Facial expression of emotion: New findings, new questions. *Psychological Science, 3*, 34-38. doi: 10.1111/j.1467-9280.1992.tb00253.x

Ekman, P. (1992c). An argument for basic emotions.*Cognition and emotion, 6*, 169 – 200. doi:10.1080/02699939208411068

Ekman, P. (1994a). Strong evidence for universals in facial expressions: A reply to Russell's mistaken critique. *Psychologicall Bulletin*, 115, 268-287.

Ekman, P. (1994b). All emotions are basic. In: P. Ekman & R.J. Davidson (Eds). *The nature of emotion: Fundamental questions.* New York: Oxford University Press.

Ekman, P. (1999). Basic emotions. In T. Dalgleish, & M. Power (Eds.), *Handbook of cognition and emotion.* New York: Wiley.

Ekman, P., Friesen, W. V., O'Sullivan, M., Chan, A., Diacoyanni-Tarlatzis, I., Heider, K., Krause, R., Leeompte, W. A., Pitcairn, T., Ricci-Bitti, P. E., Scherer. K., Tomita, M. & Tzavaras, A. (1987). Universals and cultural differences in the judgments of facial expressions of emotion. *Journal of Personality and Social Psychology, 53*, 712-717. doi: 10.1037/0022-3514.53.4.712

Elfenbein, H. A., Mandal, M. K., Ambady, N., Harizuka, S. & Kumar, S. (2002). Cross-cultural patterns in emotion recognition: Highlighting design and analytical techniques. *Emotion, 2*(1), 75-84. doi: 10.1037/1528-3542.2.1.75

Enfield, S., Tonge, B.,Turner, G., Parmenter, T., & Smith, A. (1999).Longitudinal course of behavioural and emotional problems of young persons with Prader-Willi, Fragile X, Williams and Dwon syndrome. *Journal of intellectual and Development Disability, 24* (4): 349-354. Retrieved from http://www.deepdyve.com/lp/informa-healthcare/longitudinal-course-of-behavioural-and-emotional-problems-of-young-bo1ncj00nf

English, H. B. (1924). Emotion as related to instinct. *Psychological Bulletin, 21*(6), 309-326. doi: 10.1037/h0069078

Freeman, S. F. N. & Kasari, C. (*2002*) Characteristics and Qualities of the Play Dates of Children With Down Syndrome: Emerging or True Friendships? *American Journal on Mental Retardation*, *107*(1), 16-31.

Fridlund, A. J. (1994). *Human facial expressions: An evolutionary view*. New York: Academic Press.

Fridlund, A. J. (1997). The new ethology of human facial expression. In J. A. Russell & J. M. Fernández-Dols (Eds.), *The psychology of facial expression* (pp. 103 –129). Cambridge, UK: Cambridge University Press.

Geoffrey, R., Argus, P. C., Terry, P. B. & Dinsdale, S. L. (2004). Measurement of mood in adolescents with intellectual disability. *Research in Developmental Disabilities*, *25*(6), 493-507. Retrieved from http://dx.doi.org/10.1016/j.ridd.2004.05.001

Gray, J. A. (1982). *The neuropsychology of anxiety*. Oxford, UK: Oxford University Press.

Gross, J. J. (Ed.) (2007). *Handbook of emotion regulation*. New York: Guilford

Gruber, J., Oveis, C., Keltner, D. & Johnson, S. L. (2011). A discrete emotions approach to positive emotion disturbance in depression. *Cognition & Emotion*, 25(1), 40-52. doi: 10.1080/02699931003615984.

Gyurak, A., Goodkind, M. S., Kramer, J. H., Miller, B. L. & Levenson, R. W. (2012). Executive functions and the down-regulation and up-regulation of emotion *Cognition & Emotion, 26*(1), 103-118. doi: 10.1080/02699931.2011.557291

Hodapp, R. M., DesJardin, J. L. & Ricci, L. A. (2003). Genetic syndromes of mental retardation: should they matter for the early interventionist? *Infants and Young Children, 16*(2), 152-160. Retrieved from http://depts.washington.edu/isei/iyc/hodapp_16_2.pdf

Izard, C. E. (2007a). Emotion Feelings Stem from Evolution and Neurobiological Development, Not From Conceptual Acts: Corrections for Barrett et al. (2007). *Perspectives on Psychological Science,* 2(4), 404-405. doi: 10.1111/j.1745-6916.2007.00053.x

Izard, C. E. (2007b). Basic Emotions, Natural Kinds, Emotion Schemas, and a New Paradigm. *Perspectives on Psychological Science, 2*(3), 260-280. doi: 10.1111/j.1745-6916.2007.00044.x

Izard, C. E. (1977). *Human emotions*. New York: Plenum Press.

Izard, C. E. (2009). Emotion Theory and Research: Highlights, Unanswered Questions, and Emerging Issues. *Annu. Rev. Psychol. 60*:1–25. doi: 10.1146/annurev.psych.60.110707.163539

Izard, C. E. (2009). Emotion Theory and Research: Highlights, Unanswered Questions, and Emerging Issues. *Annu. Rev. Psychol, 60*, 1–25. doi: 10.1146/annurev.psych.60.110707.163539

Izard, C. E. (1971). *The Face of Emotion.* New York: Appleton-Century-Crofts

Izard, C. E. (1992). Basic Emotions, Relations Among Emotions, and Emotion-Cognition Relations. *Psychological Review, 99*(3), 561-565. doi: 10.1037/0033-295X.99.3.561

Izard, C. E. (2007a). Basic emotions, natural kinds, emotion schemas, and a new paradigm. *Personal. Psychol. Sci.* 2:260–80.

Izard, C. E. (2010). The many meanings/aspects of emotion: Definitions, functions, activation, and regulation. *Emotion Review*, 2, 363-370. doi: 10.1177/1754073910374661

Izard, C. E., Fantauzzo, C. A., Castle, J. M., Haynes, O. M., Rayias, M. F. & Putnam, P. H. (1995). The ontogeny and significance of infants' facial expressions in the first 9 months of life. *Dev. Psychol.* 31:997–1013. Retrieved from http://psycnet.apa.org/index.cfm?fa=buy.optionToBuy&id=1996-13989-001

Izard, C. E. (1994). Innate and Universal Facial Expressions: Evidence From Developmental and Cross-Cultural Research. *Psychological Bulletin, 115*(2), 288-299. doi: 10.1037/0033-2909.115.2.288

Jahromi, L. B., Gulsrud, A. & Kasari, C. (2008). Emotional Competence in Children With Down Syndrome: Negativity and Regulation. *American Journal on Mental Retardation. 113*(1), 32-43.doi: 10.1352/0895-8017(2008)113[32:ECICWD]2.0.CO;2

James, W. (1884). What is an emotion, *Mind, 9,* 188-205.Retrieved from http://psychclassics.yorku.ca/author.htm

Jeringan, T. L., Bellugi, U., & Sowell, E. (1993). Cerebral morphological distinctions between William's and Down's syndromes. *Archives of Neurology, 50*(2), 186-191. Retrieved from http://lcn.salk.edu/publications/1993/Jernigan%20-%20Cerebral%20Morphologic%20Distinctions%201993.pdf

Kasari, C. & Freeman, S. (2001). Task-related social behaviour in children with Down syndrome. American Journal on Mental Retardation, 106(3), 253–264.

Kasari, C. & Sigman, M. (1996). Expression and understanding of emotion in atypical development: Autism and Down syndrome. In M. Lewis & M.W. Sullivan (Eds.), *Emotional development in atypical children* (pp. 109-130) Mahwah, NJ: Erlbaum.

Kasari, C., Mundy, P., Yirmiya, N. & Sigman, M. (1990). Affect and attention in children with Down syndrome. *American Journal on Mental Retardation, 95*, 55-67.

Keltner, D., Ekman, P., Gonzaga, G. C. & Beer, J. (2003). Facial expression of emotion. In: Davidson, Richard J., Scherer, Klaus R., Goldsmith, H. Hill (Eds.), *Handbook of Affective Sciences*(1st ed.). New York: Oxford University Press

Kleinginna, P. R. & Kleinginna, A. M. (1981). A categorized list of emotion definitions, with suggestions for a consensual definition. *Motivat. Emot. 5*, 345_/379. Retrieved from http://148.202.18.157/sitios/catedrasnacionales/material/2010b/sanz/kleinginna1981.pdf

Kopp, C. B., Krakow, J. B. & Johnson, K. L. (1983). Strategy production by young Down syndrome children. *American Journal of Mental Deficiency 88*:164–169.

Lench, H. C. Flores, S. A. & Bench, S. W. (2011). Discrete emotions predict changes in cognition, judgment, experience, behaviour, and physiology: A meta-analysis of experimental emotion elicitations. *Psychological Bulletin, 137*(5), 834-855. doi: 10.1037/a0024244

Lichtenstein-Vidne, L., Henik, A. & Safadi, Z. (2012). Task relevance modulates processing of distracting emotional stimuli. *Cognition & Emotion, 26*(1), 42-52. doi: 10.1080/02699931.2011.567055

Lubec, G. (2003). The brain in Down syndrome (trisomy 21). Retrieved from http://altonweb.com/cs/downsyndrome/lubec.html

Lundquvist. D. &Öhman, A. (2005). Caught by the evil eye: Nonconscious information processing, emotion and attention to facial stimuli. In: Lisa F. Barret, Paula M.

Niedenthal & PiotrWinkielman (Eds.), *Emotion and consciousness*. (pp.97-122). New York: Guilford Press.

Mans, L., Cicchetti, D. & Sroufe, L. A. (1978). Mirror reactions of Down's syndrome infants and toddlers: Cognitive underpinnings of self- recognition. *Child Development, 49*, 1247-1250. Retrieved from http://www.jstor.org/discover/10.2307/1128771?uid=3737952&uid=2129&uid=2&uid=70&uid=4&sid=21101486986083

Merker , B. (2007). Consciousness without a cerbral cortex: A challenge for neuroscience and medicine. *Behavioural and Brain Sciences*, 30(1), 63-81.

Morales, M. G. E. & Lopez, R. E. O. (2005). Mecanismos cognitivos de reconocimiento de información emocional en personas con síndrome de Down. *Revista Médica Internacional sobre Síndrome de Down, 9*(1), 2-6. Retrieved from http://www.google.es/url?sa=t&rct=j&q=mecanismos%20cognitivos%20de%20reconocimiento%20de%20información%20emocional%20en%20personas%20con%20s%C3%ADndrome%20de%20down&source=web&cd=1&ved=0CDUQFjAA&url=http%3A%2F%2Fwww.fcsd.org%2Fmecanismos-cognitivos-de-reconocimiento-de-informaci%25C3%25B3n-emocional-facial-en-personas-con-s%25C3%25ADndrome-de-down_33158.pdf%3Fdisposition%3Dattachment&ei=TLfgUJ47yqeEB6aggIAG&usg=AFQjCNHMPNmD-So3tH6JU8vorCpsu1TqCw&bvm=bv.1355534169,d.ZG4

Morales, M. G. E. & Lopez, R. E. O. (2006). *El síndrome de Down y su mundo emocional*. México: Trillas.

Morales, M. G. E. & Lopez, R. E. O. (2010). Down syndrome and automatic processing of familiar and unfamiliar emotional faces. *International Journal of Special Education, 25(3),* 17-23. Retrieved from http://www.eric.ed.gov/ERICWebPortal/search/recordDetails.jsp?ERICExtSearch_SearchValue_0=EJ909032&searchtype=keyword&ERICExtSearch_SearchType_0=no&_pageLabel=RecordDetails&accno=EJ909032&_nfls=false&source=ae

Morales, M. G. E. & Lopez, R. E. O. (2012). Down syndrome and emotional face recognition from a connectionist point of view. *Revista Mexicana de Psicología Educativa (RMPE), 1*(2), 41-53

Morales, M. G. E., & Lopez, R. E. O. (2006). *El síndrome de Down y su mundo emocional*. México: Trillas.

Morales, M. G. E. & Lopez, R. E. O. (2011). El reconocimiento facial emocional en el síndrome de Down: modelando desde una perspectiva conexionista. *Revista Mexicana de Psicología Educativa, 1*(2), 41-53.

Morales, M. G. (2010). Nuevas direcciones metodológicas desde una visión cognitiva y neurocomputacional en la exploración del reconocimiento facial de la emoción en el síndrome de Down [New methodological approaches since a cognitive and neurocomputational view to exploring emotional facial recognition in Down syndrome]. Unpublished doctoral thesis. Universidad Autónoma de Nuevo Leon, Monterrey, México.

Morales, M. G. E., Charles, C. D. J., Castro, C. C., Lopez, R. E. O. & Mullet, E. (2012). Blame judgements among persons with Down's syndrome. Unpublished document.

Morales, M. G. E., Lopez, R. E. O. & Hedlefs, A. M. I. (2010). La psicología de las emociones: *La expresión facial como una revelación de la emoción y el pensamiento*. México: Trillas.

Mundy, P., Sigman, M. & Kasari, C. (1990). A longitudinal study of joint attention and language development in autistic children. *Journal of Autism and Developmental Disorders, 20*, 115-129. doi: 10.1007/BF02206861

Murphy, G. L. (2002). *The big book of concepts*. Cambridge, Massachussets: MIT Press.

Oatley, K. (2004). *Emotions: A brief history*. USA: Blackwell Publishing

Ortony, A. & Turner, T. J. (1990). What's Basic About Basic Emotions? *Psychological Review, 97*(3), 315-331. doi: 10.1037/0033-295X.97.3.315

Ortony, A., Clore, G. & Collins, A. (1988). *The cognitive structure of emotions*. Cambridge: Cambridge University Press

Pace, B., Lynm, C. & Glass, R. (2001). Down syndrome, *JAMA*. Retrieved from http://www.hmc.psu.edu/healthinfo/articles/downsyndrome.pdf

Pankseepp, J. (1998). *Affective neuroscience: The foundations of human and animal emotions*. New York: Oxford University Press.

Panksepp, J. (2007). Neurologizing the Psychology of Affects: How Appraisal-Based Constructivism and Basic Emotion Theory Can Coexist. *Perspectives on Psychological Science, 2* (3), 281-296.doi. 10.1111/j.1745-6916.2007.00045.x

Panksepp, J. (2005). On the embodied neural nature of core emotional affects. *Journal of Consciousness Studies, 12*, 158–184. Retrieved from http://www.ncbi.nlm.nih.gov/pmc/articles/PMC3181986/

Parrott, W. (2001). Emotions in Social Psychology, Psychology Press, Philadelphia

Pennington, B., Moon, J., Edgin, J., Stedron, J. & Nade, L. (2003). The neuropsychology of Down syndrome: evidence for hippocampal disfunction. *Child Development, 74*(1), 75-93. doi: 10.1111/1467-8624.00522

Pitcairn, T. K. & Wishart, J. G. (1994). Reactions of young children with Down's syndrome to an impossible task. *British Journal of Developmental Psychology. 12*(4), 485-489. doi: 10.1111/j.2044-835X.1994.tb00649.x

Pitcairn, T. & Wishart, J. (2000). Face processing in Children With Down Syndrome. En D. Weeks, R. Chua & D. Elliot (Eds.*). Perceptual-Motor behaviour in Down syndrome* (pp. 123-147). Edinburgh, Inglaterra: Human Kinetics.

Plutchik, R. (1994). *The psychology and biology of emotion*. Nueva York, NY, EE. UU.: Harper Collins College Publishers.

Plutchik, R. (2001). The Nature of Emotions: Human emotions have deep evolutionary roots, a fact that may explain their complexity and provide tools for clinical practice. *American Scientist, 89*(4), 344-350. doi: 10.1511/2001.4.344

Poirel, N., Cassotti, M., Beaucousin, V., Pineau, A. & Houdé, O. (2012). Pleasant emotional induction broadens the visual world of young children. *Cognition & Emotion, 26*(1), 186-191. doi: 10.1080/02699931.2011.589430.

Ponari, M., Conson, M., D'Amico, N. P., Grossi, D. & Trojano, L. (2012). Mapping correspondence between facial mimicry and emotion recognition in healthy subjects. *Emotion, 12*(6), 1398-1403. doi:10.1037/a0028588

Power, M. & Dalgleish, T. (2008). *Cognition and Emotion: From order to disorder (2nd ed.)*. Hove and New York: Psychology Press.

Raz, N., Torres, I. & Briggs, S. D. (1995). Selective neuroanatomical abnormalities in Down's syndrome and their cognitive correlates: Evidence from MRI morphometry. *Neurology, 45*, 356-366. Retrieved from http://www.neurology.org/content/45/2/356

Reddy, V., Williams, E. & Vaughan, A. (2001). Sharing laughter: the humour of pre-school children with Down syndrome. *Down Syndrome Research and Practice, 7*(3), 125-128. Retrieved from http://www.down-syndrome.org/reports/121/

Reddy, V., Williams, E. & Vaughan, A. (2002). Sharing humour and laughter in autism and Down's syndrome. *British Journal Psychology, 93*, 219-242. doi: 10.1348/000712602162553

Roch-Levecq, A. C. (2006). Production of basic emotions by children with congenital blindness: Evidence for the embodiment of theory of mind. *British Psychological Society, 24*(3), 507-528. doi: 10.1348/026151005X50663

Roizen, N. & Patterson, D. (2003). Down's syndrome. *The lancet, 361*, 1281-1289. doi:10.1016/S0140-6736(03)12987-X

Rosner, B. A., Hodapp, R. M., Fidler, D. J., Sagun, J. N. & Dykens, E. M. (2004). Social competence in persons with Prader-Willi, Williams and Down syndromes. *Journal of Applied Research in Intellectual Disabilities,* 17, 209-217. doi: 10.1111/j.1468-3148.2004.00200.x

Russell, J. A. & Bullock, M. (1986). On the dimensions preschoolers use to interpret facial expression of emotion. *Developmental Psychology, 22* (1), 97-102. doi: 10.1037/0012-1649.22.1.97

Russell, J. A. (1980). A Cirumplex Model of Affect. *Journal of Personality and Social Psychology, 39*, 1161-1178. Retrieved from https://www2.bc.edu/~russeljm/publications/Russell1980.pdf

Russell, J. A. (2003). [Image] Retrieved on February 27, 2008, from http://www2.bc.edu/~russeljm/

Sabini, J. & Silver, M. (2005). Ekman's basic emotions: Why not love and jealousy?.*Cognition and Emotion, 19*(5), 693-712.DOI:10.1080/02699930441000481

Sapolsky, R. M. (2007). Stress, stress-related disease, and emotion regulation. In J. J. Gross (Ed.), *Handbook of emotion regulation* (pp. 606–615). New York: Guilford

Schachter, S. & Singer, J. E. (1962). Cognitive, social, and physiological determinants of emotional state. *Psychological Review, 69*, 379–399. doi: 10.1037/h0046234

Serafica, F. C. & Cicchetti, D. (1976). Down's syndrome children in the Strange Situation: Attachment and exploratory behaviours. *Merrill-Palmer Quarterly, 21,* 137- 150.

Shariff, A. F. & Tracy, J. L. (2011). What Are Emotion Expressions For? *Current Directions in Psychological Science, 20*(6), 395-399. doi: 10.1177/0963721411424739.

Shaver, P. R. & Mikulincer, M. (2007). Adult attachment strategies and the regulation of emotion. In J. J. Gross (Ed.), *Handbook of emotion regulation* (pp. 446-465). New York: Guilford Press.

Slatcher, R. B. & Trentacosta, C. J. (2011). A naturalistic observation study of the links between parental depressive symptoms and preschoolers behaviours in everyday life. Journal of Family Psychology, 25, 444-448. Retrieved from http://www.richslatcher.com/papers/SlatcherTrentacosta_EARdepression_JFP_2011.pdf

Smith, M. C. & Dodson, D. G. (1996). Facial expression *Journal of Abnormal Psychology, 105*(4), 602-608. doi: 10.1037/0021-843X.105.4.602

Smith, M. & Walden, T. (1998, agosto). *Emotion regulation in children with Down syndrome*. Documento presentado en la American Psychological Association Annual Convetion, San Fracisco, CA, EE. UU.

Sroufe, A. (1998). *Desarrollo emocional: la organización de la vida emocional en los primeros años*. México, D.F.: Oxford University Press.

Stratford, B. (1998). *Síndrome de Down: pasado, presente y futuro*. México: Edivision.

Stearns, P. N. (2008). History of emotions: Issues of change and impact. In M. Lewis, J. M. Haviland-Jones & L. F. Barrett (Eds.), *Handbook of emotions*. (3rd ed., pp. 17-31) Guilford Press.

Stets, J. E. & Turner, J. H. (2008). The sociology of emotions. In M. Lewis, J. M. Haviland-Jones & L. F. Barrett (Eds.), *Handbook of emotions*. (3rd ed., pp. 32-46) Guilford Press.

Strongman, K. T. (2003). The psychology of emotion: the everyday life to theory. England: John Wiley & SonsLtd.

Thompson, J. (1990). *Ideology and modern culture: critical social theory in the era of mass communication*. Carnbridge: Polity Press

Thompson, R. A., Cicchetti, D., Lamb, M. E. & Malkin, C. (1985). Emotional responses of Down syndrome and normal infants in the Strange Situation: The organization of affective behaviour in infants. *Developmental Psychology, 21*(5), 828-841. doi: 10.1037/0012-1649.21.5.828

Toffolo, M. B. J., Smeets, M. A. M. & van den Hout, M. A. (2012). Proust revisited: Odours as triggers of aversive memories. *Cognition & Emotion, 26*(1), 83-92. doi: 10.1080/02699931.2011.555475.

Turk, J. & Cornish, K. (1998). Face recognition and emotion perception in boys with Fragile X syndrome. *Journal of Intellectual Disability Research, 42*(6), 490-499.

Virji-Babul, N., Moiseev, A., Cheung, T., Cheyne, D., Ribary, U. & Weeks, D. (2012). Adults with Down syndrome show right hemisphere dominance during right-handed voluntary movements. Retrieved fromhttp://www.dsrf.org/research/research-projects/

vonSalisch, M. (2001). Children's emotional development: Challenges in their relationship to parents, peer, and friends. *International Journal of Behavioural Development, 25*(4), 310-319. doi: 10.1080/01650250143000058

Watson, D. & Tellegen, A. (1985). Towards a consensual structure of mood. *Psychological Bulletin*, 98, 219-235.doi: 10.1037/0033-

Watson, J. B. (1916). Behaviour and the concept of mental disease. Retrieved on April 12, 2008, from http://philpapers.org/rec/WATBAT

Widen, S. C. & Russell, J. A. (2010). Descriptive and Prescriptive Definitions of Emotion. *Emotion Review, 2*(4) 377-378. doi: 10.1177/1754073910374667

Wishart, J. & Pitcairn, T. (2000). Recognition of identity and expression in faces by children with Down syndrome. *American Journal on Mental Retardation, 105*(6), 466-479. Retrieved from http://www.aaiddjournals.org/doi/abs/10.1352/0895-8017%282005%29110%5B378%3AERBCWD%5D2.0.CO%3B2

Wranik, T., Barrett, L. F. & Salovey, P. (2007). Intelligent emotion regulation: Is knowledge power? In J. Gross (Ed.), *Handbook of emotion regulation* (pp. 393-407). New York: Guilford.

Wuerker, A. M. (1996). Communication patterns and expressed emotion*Schizophrenia Bulletin, 22*(4), 671-690. Retrieved from http://schizophreniabulletin.oxfordjournals.org/content/22/4/671.full.pdf

Chapter 3

The Down Syndrome Affective Processing Style from a Facial Recognition Perspective

Abstract

Down syndrome research has mainly addressed cognitive and behavioural dimensions; it was only very recently that some scientists began to consider the emotional system of those with this genetic condition. In addition, most academic research inside this area provides an empirical data corpus from a deficit point of view rather than trying to identify the complete cognitive-emotional system functioning of a person with DS. This has strongly limited the possibility of identifying an alternative affective style typifying members from this population. In this chapter it is assumed that identification of a DS affective style can be achieved using cognitive science experimental methodology. To this purpose, some affective priming study designs to study emotional face recognition are introduced to explore the DS emotion system.

3.1. Global Remarks about Down Syndrome Brain Structure and a Possible Cognitive-Affective Processing Style

Frequently, parents, special education teachers and others report that people with DS seem to share among them a specific emotion-behaviour pattern that makes them different from the rest of us. In particular, some people think they are emotional in extreme. Take for instance the following conversation commentary from a mother of young child with DS:

> "Down syndrome children are very fickle; they can stay very happy for quite some time and suddenly they change into a sea of sadness and crying".

Other people think that they are persons with plenty of love and nobility. This can be seen from some teachers and parents' remarks about these children with DS:

"They are very loving and romantic..."
"They are incapable of harming someone else..."
"These children are extremely compassionate...."

It is not so difficult to notice a possible stereotype imposing a label of extreme emotionality over members of this population. How accurate is this? Is it possible to find an emotional phenotype that sets them apart from other typical ways to experience emotions?

First, let us remember that human emotion is a complex psychological and behavioural system that embraces aspects such as: a) Different domains (e.g. expression, regulation, experience and/or emotional processing) and b) internal variability of each emotion domain (e.g. physiological, cognitive, behavioural, etc.) which can be permanent or transitory for only one member of the group, or throughout the population. That is, a person could have a personal emotion profile but at the same time this person might share emotional standards that typify an entire population. Take for instance people with clinically diagnosed anxiety or depression, which are emotional disorders typified by a specific way of processing negative and positive information. Even though all of us are vulnerable to experiencing emotion this way, the clinical condition does not typify all of us as emotional beings. An interesting question arises from this observation: Is this particular vs. global emotional difference the same for people with DS?

In order to deal with this question is necessary first to introduce a brief review on the concept of affective style, including its components and underlying variables. We will then use this commentary to frame emotional processing styles inside the DS field.

3.1.1. Affective Style: Definition, Variables and Components

Since early stages of our life, all of us begin to show individual differences on the way we experience and express emotions (Oveis, Gruber, Keltner, Stamper & Boyce, 2009). This is also the case for people with DS. They can present differences regarding the intensity and quality of an emotion over a single object or event. Take for instance the following answers from an interview to two teenagers with DS:

Interviewer: How would you feel if somebody hit you?
Teenager A with DS: I would not forgive him; it is wrong. The other day "Mr. X" hit me and I got angry. I do not talk to him anymore.
Teenager B with DS: Let me tell you, the other day Mr. "X" and Mr. "Y" got into fist fight. I really do not like that they fight each other. Particularly, I do not like somebody hitting me.
Interviewer: Then, how would you feel if somebody hits you?
Teenager B with DS: Bad, sad. Then it will pass over.

Even when both answers share the same negative valence, their intentions represent different emotional goals. That is, the emotional reactivity is the same, but they do not manifest the same emotional pursuit and thus depending on the context the same event might lead to different behavioural concerns.

Because of this, a concern emerges about the possibility of finding an emotional profile typifying a group of persons (e.g. a DS emotional profile). To this respect, there is some academic evidence suggesting that peoples' emotional differences can be genetically constrained (Hamann & Canli, 2004; también véase Lesch, Bengel, Heils, Sabol, Greenberg, Petri, Benjamin, Muller, Hamer, Murphy, 1996). Thus, since Down syndrome is a genetic condition that typifies variability of an entire population then it can be hypothesized that a possible specific emotional profile or a specific affective style is developed due to genetic constraints.

The idea of specific processing patterns of emotional information is not new. At the end of the 1960s, Ehrlich and Lipsey identified a new perception variable they named affective style and defined as "an individual's characteristic mode of affective response to people in first encounters". Collateral academic efforts on this direction emerged from the neuroscience field that define affective style as systematic and stable physiological processing underlying emotional regulation and emotional reactivity through individual variation (Davidson, 1998). Research inside this field has centered on exploring the functioning of at least five affective style components: a) people's capacity to detect and to react to the same emotional stimulus (response threshold), b) emotional response to a stimulus intensity or magnitude (known as response peak) and c) individual differences concerning emotional response time (the rise time to a emotional response peak, the recovery time and response time duration). People's different reaction times to these variables relate to emotional valence-specific features of emotional reactivity or affective responses (Davidson, 1998, 2003, 2004).

To put these affective style concepts into perspective, let us introduce the case for sensation of pain and DS. Apparently, emotional reactivity (intensity, amplitude, and threshold) to aversive stimuli from this population is different from a typical one. For example, a research study reported verbal reports of pain of infants with and without DS showed that typical infants required less aversive stimulation to elicit crying behaviour (Lind, Vuorenkoski, Rosberg, Paratanen, Wasz-Hockert, 1970). However, this reactivity difference to pain among populations is not maintained through all the range of instances of possible negative dimension. Moreover, reactivity threshold differences to the same negative stimulus can be obtained among members from the population with DS.

Another relevant aspect to consider about an affective style is the emotion regulation process. This process relates to a wide range of emotional challenges, disposition moods and relevant cognitive processing (Davidson, 1998). Regarding DS, not much is known about emotional regulation but some initial research suggests differences between this population and a typical population (see chapter 2). These emotion regulation processes are assumed to be relevant because they delimit vulnerability and resilience capacity (Davidson, 1998). That is, some affective styles are better than others in dealing with emotional experiences (Hofmann & Kashdan, 2010). For example, people who ruminate more than usual on events happening to them, seem to develop prolonged negative mood states that frequently lead them toward an emotional disorder (e.g. depression; Papageorgiou & Wells, 2004). On the other side, people who practice emotional acceptance seem to be more resilient and have better stress management when they are confronted with difficult situations (e.g., Hayes, Luoma, Bond, Masuda & Lillis, 2006)

The reasons why people seem to vary their affective style are still being explored, with some research in this direction relating affective style and temperament (Kagan, Reznick & Snidman, 1988), and affective style and personality (Gross, Sutton, & Ketelaar, 1998) as well as vulnerability to psychopathology (Meehl, 1975). Additional academic efforts are being made to try to determine the neural basis of affective style and its emotional mechanisms. Take for instance some research results provided by Davidson and Irwin (1999) suggesting specific emotion physiology relating the amygdala and the prefrontal cortex to process negative and positive information (see also Davidson, 2003). This is relevant to DS in that genetically constrained neural strata of the amygdala and the prefrontal cortex have been identified. Even when this atypical brain development could be adverse, it also represents an opportunity to explore our emotional system as well as DS emotional brain. It is our strongest belief that direct or indirect determination of how our emotional brain behaves when under stress due to a genetic condition, will empower medical research to better clinical interventions and the development of a higher quality of life.

3.1.2. DS Brain Structure and Affective Style

The differences between DS brain's morphology (e.g. a defective development of frontal lobes, Lubec, 2003; Raz et al., 1995; a reduced brainstem, Benda, 1971; reduced temporal-limbic brain areas: Jeringan, Bellugi, Sowell, Doherty & Hesselink, 1993 as well as a reduced-size hippocampus, Raz et al., 1995) and that of a typical brain, play an important role on emotion information processing. For instance, some difficulties in recognizing negative information in the DS population are associated with dysfunctional functioning of the amygdala (Wishart, 2000). Nevertheless, there is still some debate about how the volume of the DS amygdala (see Jackowski, Laureano, Del'Aquilla, Monteiro de Moura, Assuncao, Silva & Saloma, 2011) affects the emotional experience in this population. Particularly, whenever they have to evaluate negative behavioural consequences such as assuming an inappropriate social distance (closeness). Here, most research on behaviour and the DS brain has taken into account three hypotheses (see also Porter, Coltheart, Langdon, 2007). The first one suggests that amygdala dysfunction is the origin for difficulty in emotion regulation and emotion recognition. The second one points to dysfunctional inhibitory mechanisms due to frontal lobe deficits. The third hypothesis speculates on the possibility of a brain tuned to process positive emotional information (the Social Salience hypothesis). The goal of this chapter is to bring attention to the first hypothesis, namely, negative recognition information due to amygdala deficits.

The amygdala dysfunction hypothesis is largely based on the idea that this neural structure is related to emotional regulation (Davidson, Putnam & Larson, 2000). Trauma or damage to typical individuals' amygdalas from accidents lead to negative information recognition deficits (e.g. Fear) (see Adolphs, Tranel & Damasio, 1998). Clinical patients with this problem will not recognize negative valence information (like anger, fear and to some extent, sadness) from sensorial modalities (auditive: emotional vocal tone, and visual: emotional facial expression; Scott et al., 1997). Interestingly, these limitations do not apply to the recognition of information related to happiness (Blair, Morris, Frith, Perrett, & Dolan, 1999). Although these emotional information processing patterns are similar to people with DS's emotion recognition deficits, there is still not enough evidence to conclude that both populations' emotional behaviours share the same amygdala physiology dysfunction. Here, a possible indirect way to bring light upon this matter is to check for similarities using demanded cognitive-emotional performance.

For example, clinical patients with amygdala damage will not be able to show an emotion system structure, as predicted by the Russell and Fehr (1987) emotion circumplex. If this cognitive-emotional limitation was presented by people with DS, it could be assumed that both populations have atypical emotional behaviour due to amygdala dysfunction. However, as already explored in the emotion circumplex pilot study from chapter 2, this is not the case for all of the people with DS. Due to variability, some of the genetically constrained persons seemed capable of achieving a circular emotional structure. At least one of the participants matched predicted typical performance. Notice that both persons were required to participate in an affective priming study requiring an emotion face recognition task. As the study showed, both participants displayed negative automatic processing recognition deficits. However, whenever they were required to recognize photos of negative faces (controlled processing) they were perfectly capable of doing it. The participant who showed a typical emotional circumplex had an IQ of 70 and was 23 years younger than another participant of 48, who had an IQ of 64. It is hard to arrive to any conclusion from this simple pilot study. However, this variability on performance is also hard to simply assign to amygdala damage. Complementary support to this observation comes from Porter et al.'s research (2007), suggesting that people with DS do not present similar emotion recognition deficits and social distance problems as those presented by clinical patients with acquired amygdala damage.

The damaged amygdala hypothesis has been increasingly relevant to emotion recognition and DS due to a research stream originating from it. These academic efforts have allowed the determination of identification and categorization difficulties in this population that are related to emotion recognition. Further research is needed to more deeply explore this atypical cognitive-functional behaviour. Another promising research field in which to deeply explore cognitive and emotional DS functioning is emotional facial recognition. This field is relevant to social interaction (Chung & Donald, 1995), and allows people to infer possible behaviours by others (Carvajal & Iglesias, 2002; Ekman, 2003; Kaiser & Wehrle, 2001). Concerns about people with DS difficulty in recognizing negative faces acknowledge that discrimination or segregation toward members of this population are based on their lack of ability to recognizing facial social disapproval, like the facial disapproval for approaching too close (Wishart & Pitcairn, 2003). To what extent this recognition dificulty applies to all members of this population is only just starting to be explored, and more research is needed, not only due to theoretical implications to emotion theory, but in order to improve the quality of life for this vulnerable population.

3.2. The Emotional Face from a Down Syndrome Point of View: Some Remarkable Scientific Findings

From the very early stages of our lives, we are capable of distinguishing emotional faces (like happiness, sadness, angry, etc) from those faces not expressing any emotion (neutral). This innate capacity is relevant because they empower us as social beings, letting us know what others think and allowing us to obtain meaningful inferences about our own consciousness as well as others (Morales et al., 2010).

Emotional face recognition research regarding ID is in the initial stages. Most research on this matter has centered on autism and similar groups' etiologies (e.g., van der Geest, Kemner, Verbaten & van Engeland, 2002). Regarding DS, emotion face recognition is just beginning and only a few set of studies on this topic are available (e.g., Annaz, Karmiloff-Smith, Johnson & Thomas, 2009; Porter, Coltheart & Langdon, 2007; Turk & Cornish, 1998; Wishart & Pitcairn, 2000; Wishart et al., 2007). In these studies, emotion face recognition ability has focused mainly on young people and infants. Take for example studies by Wishart and Pitcairn (2000) to test children with DS's capacity to recognize emotion face recognition. The first study required a sample of young people with an age range between 8 and 14 years old to perform two experimental tasks: to match people by age groups, and to match an emotion facial expression with a short story. Their performance was compared and matched by age against a sample composed of typical individuals of similar age. Even though some the group with DS tested as being slower to classify faces to age groups, they generally had similar performance as the typical persons' group. However, they had a significant poorer performance classifying emotions, particularly emotions like fear and surprise.

Similar results were obtained in another study by Wishart et al. (2007) where emotion face recognition capacity was explored using different groups with or without ID (X fragile syndrome, DS, non specified ID and typical children with equivalent cognitive and linguistic abilities). In this study, one task was to test basic facial processing abilities using an identity matching task. In another study task, the same participants had to match emotional stimuli (happiness, sadness, anger, surprise, fear and disgust). Results showed that participants with DS seem to have the same ability to recognize facial identity as other children with different ID etiologies (X fragile syndrome and non-specified ID) and typical children. Again, whenever it comes to emotion facial recognition, members of the population with ID performed more poorly, particuarly participants with DS, who showed difficulties in recognizing fear. Additional research confirms that study participants with DS have difficulties in recognizing negative facial information (Turk & Cornish, 1998), suggesting that brain functioning under this genetic condition is typified by a specific negative information processing style (Conrad, Schmidt, Niccols, Polak, Riniolo & Burack, 2007).

Overall, the above academic evidence strongly suggests that people with DS have difficulties in processing facial information (Williams, Wishart, Pitcairn & Willis, 2005; Wishart, Cebula, Willis & Pitcairn, 2007; Pitcairn & Wishart, 2000; Turk & Cornish, 1998; Wishart & Pitcairn, 2000) particularly negative facial information (Wishart & Pitcairn, 2000).

Curiosity about the specific cognitive nature underlying this constrained way in which they experience emotion has brought new scientific attention from the cognitive science field. These new academic insights are described next.

3.3. Opening the Down Syndrome's Emotional Black Box with a Cognitive Key

A cognitive view of human emotion assumes that every emotion has a rational component that includes automatic cognitive appraisals as well as controlled processes, and this processing occupies an important place on timeline elicitation. Here, the sequence of events by which an emotional response is elicited has been the object of academic analysis from a number of theoretical points of view (see Figure 3.1).

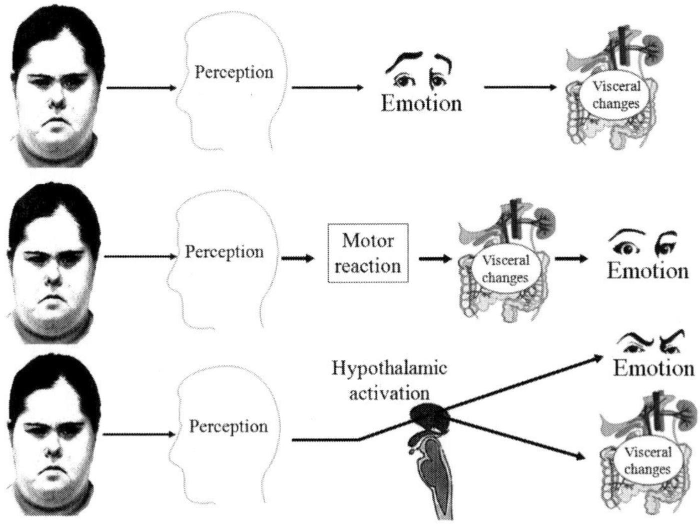

Figure 3.1. Different theoretical views (see text) have explored the sequence of physical and mental events occurring inside the timeline in which an emotion is elicited (inspired in Plutchik, 1994).

The examples shown in Figure 3.1. first describe (top) a commonsense view of emotion elicitation. Here it is assumed that once an event or object is perceived, this will activate a specific emotion that will lead to a corporal change, one that is consciously experienced by a person (feeling an emotion). Contrary to this view (center), the William James-Lange model assumes that once a stimulus is perceived motor and visceral changes will elicit the emotion experienced. Finally (bottom), the Cannon-Bard model suggests that after perceiving a stimulus, thalamic processing will produce parallel activation of visceral changes and a corresponding emotion experience (Plutchick, 1994). Notice that no matter the kind of model, stimulus perception comes first inside the emotion activation timeline. It is precisely this "perception" that implies a myriad of complex neural processes and intervention of sophisticated cognitive appraisal mechanisms happening in a matter of milliseconds, that allows a person to decide if a given event has positive or negative connotation.

This incredibly fast initial emotional appraisal system has been object of academic analysis. The research field in charge of exploring the system goes under the name of "appraisal theories of emotion". Next, we will describe some relevant theoretical developments from this field in order to understand more about the emotional system of people with DS.

3.3.1. Appraisal Theories of Emotion and Down Syndrome

Basically, appraisal theories of emotion explore those cognitive mechanisms involved in evaluating the emotional content of stimuli from the very early stages of cognitive processing (see Schorr, 2001). A seminal work on this direction in current theory is presented by Lazarus (2000, 2001), which assumes that a very fast sequence of evaluations from a stimulus is needed before a person decides on its emotional significance. These evaluations are not necessarily conscious, and this appraisal processing explains why different people can emotionally react in different ways to the same event or object. In addition, this system also explains why a person is able to emotionally react differently at different times, to the same object.

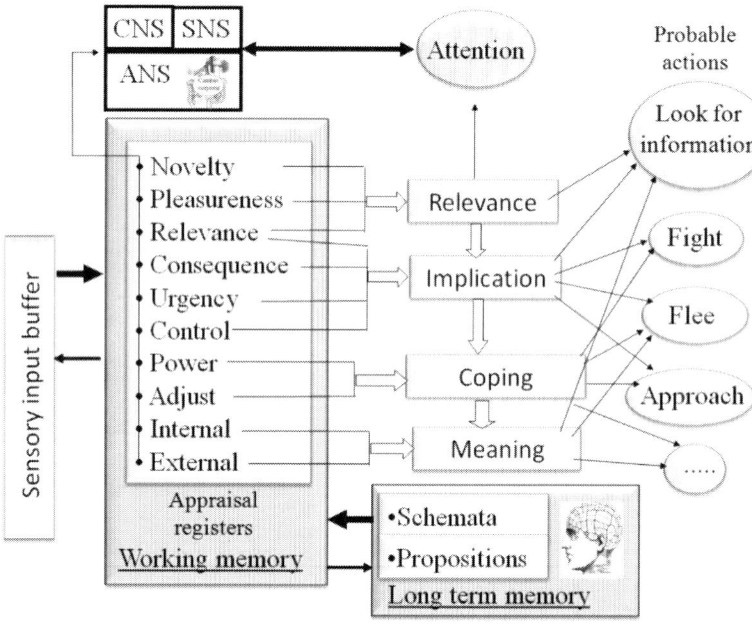

Figure 3.2. A processing model of emotion (multilevel sequential checking) that implies physical reactions by the Central Nervous System (CNS), the Autonomous Nervous System (ANS) and the Somatic Nervous System (SNS) to provide physiological support to cognitive processing components involved in sequential appraisals of a stimulus.

Another representative emotion appraisal model, entitled Multilevel Sequential Checking (also known as The Component Process Model CPM) has been presented by Scherer (1987, 2001). This model describes how low-level cognitive appraisals trigger bodily reactions, subjective feelings and specific behaviours associated with emotional experiences. In doing so, the participation of a human processing model is used to specify cognitive processing parameters necessary to guide attention, as well as other cognitive architecture (see Figure 3.2). For example, on assigning stimulus relevance, it is necessary to identify the participation of specific attention and memory processes, in order to determine possible immediate danger and a possible immediate behavioural response (Fight, flee or freeze).

Note from this processing model that short term memory processing as well as attention processing are goal oriented mechanisms providing necessary information in each evaluation step. This is possible because very fast parallel processing of information (short term memory parameter processing) about an environmental stimulus (for novelty, consequence, relevance, etc) then enables judgment for possible emotional reactions that lead to specific adaptive behaviours (Bargh, 1999; Gutierrez, 2006; Morales, 2004; Morales & Lopez, 2005). Thus, exploring how the recognition of an emotional face leads to psychological and physical/behavioural consequences, demands powerful research methodology in order to identify cognitive parameter processing.

Recently, a new experimental paradigm with the name Affective Priming has emerged to empower emotion scientists to deal with required experimental demands to explore emotion appraisal processing. In particular, this methodological approach has been useful to explore how people's appraisal mechanisms change through time as well as to study personal differences on emotional appraisal (Morales & Lopez, 2006). Specifically, the successful achievements coming from this cognitive method are based on the possibility of determining how emotional memory information affects recognizing the emotion content of environmental information (Musch & Klauer, 2003; also remember Bowers' emotion inhibitory mechanisms from chapter 2). Thus, a typical affective priming study identifies how the emotional valence of a stimulus (prime) affects the recognition of another stimulus' (target) emotional valence (Fazio, 1995). Here, a classic experiment task requires to the study participants to decide on the target valence, that is, if the target is positive, negative or neutral. An experimental events sequence defined in this kind of studies is presented in Figure 3.3.

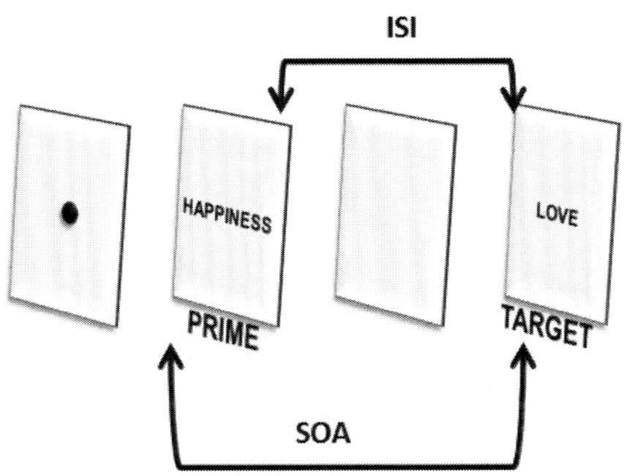

Figure 3.3. The experimental events sequence from a typical affective priming study. Here, the presentation of stimuli (both prime and target) is mediated by two time parameters: An Inter Stimulus Interval (ISI) time parameter (time between the prime and target) and a Stimulus Onset Asynchrony (SOA) time parameter (time elapsed between prime and target onsets).

An affective priming experimental sequence normally begins by first centering the participant's gaze at the computer screen center (by presenting a centered dot). Then after this centered stimulus is erased, the prime appears (a possible negative, positive, or neutral stimulus) and the study participant has to silently read it. After the prime is erased, the target is presented and the participant has to decide by selecting positive, negative or neutral on a computer keyboard, to indicated the target's emotional content. It is known that response time is faster if prime and target are emotionally congruent (positive-positive, negative-negative) than it is if they are incongruent (positive-negative, neutral-positive, neutral-negative) or if only neutral. On the other hand, experimental manipulation of the ISI and the SOA will induce either cognitive automatic processing, or controlled processing. Affective behaviour in which the presentation of an emotional stimulus may facilitate or interfere with the emotional recognition of a second one is called the affective priming effect (Musch, and Klauer, 2003; Fazio, 1995; Fazio, Sanbonmatsu, Powell and Kardes, 1986).

The affective priming effect has been recognized in reaction to a great diversity of stimuli such as pictures of animals, odors, drawings, etc. (see De Houwer, Hermans & Eelen, 1998; Hermans, Bayens & Eelen, 1998; Giner, Sorolla, García & Bargh, 1999). Among the strongest affective priming effects are visual stimuli (Dimberg, Thunberg & Elmehed, 2000; Fiedler, 2003; Gutierrez, 2006). In particular, emotional faces stimuli, since this visual information has ecological validity due to its relevance to social interaction and social communication (Harwood, Hall, Schinkfield & Alison, 1999). Moreover, facial stimuli are very helpful to people who for some reason are not capable of reading, such as some people with ID.

The affective priming technique has been used to explore emotional phenomena through a wide sample set of populations, including adults, teenagers and children, with or without emotional disorders (e.g., Lopez, 2009; Morales, Lopez & Hedlefs, 2010; Musch & Klauer, 2003; Parrish, 2007). However, it has not been until recently that this experimental paradigm has been used to explore people with DS´ emotional system. Seminal and intriguing results in this line of research are described next.

3.3.2. Down Syndrome's Automatic Processing of Emotional Facial Information through the Affective Priming Paradigm

Emotional and non-emotional facial recognition research is typified by the use of tests requiring some face recognition task (Matsumoto, LeRoux, Wilson-Cohn, Raroque, Kooken, Ekman, Yizarry, Loewinger, Uchida, Yee, Amo & Coh, 2000) or computerized reaction time in face recognition tasks (e.g., Calder, 2003; Morales, Charles & Lopez, 2008; Pollak & Kistler, 2002).

The main research technique in the exploration of people with DS's abilities to face recognition has been through standardized facial recognition tests. Although valuable information is obtained using this approach, there hasn't been much attention payed to a potentially useful alternative: the Human Information Processing (HIP) approach. The research benefits of using HIP methodology (like affective priming) offer a new, complementary and insightful way to support or reject previous traditional ways of studying facial recognition in this population.

Seminal affective priming research testing emotional face recognition abilities in persons with DS has already been conducted by Morales and Lopez (2005, 2006, 2010, and 2011). Take for instance a pilot study from these authors (Morales, 2004; Morales & Lopez, 2005), in which four participants with DS were tested on their ability to classify emotional faces (positive and negative) and non emotional faces using an affective priming approach. As expected, these participants presented difficulties in recognizing negative information even through automatic processing. It is important to notice this study included facial stimuli that were from a different cultural context (emotional faces were obtained from Ekman, Freisen & Hager, 2002). This might have affected recognition thresholds (a familiarity factor Kelly, Quinn, Slater, Lee, Gibson, Smith, Ge & Pascalis, 2005). When participants in a second study (Morales, 2004; Morales & Lopez, 2005) were provided facial information from their own cultural context, the participants from the first study did not present deficits in automatic processing recognition of negative facial information. At that point, the possibility of considering different emotional face recognition mechanisms emerged. However, due to the relatively small sample size from these initial studies, more research was conducted, increasing the sample size to 60 participants. Here, 20 participants with DS (experimental group; 9 women and 11 men) with an age range between 15 and 48 (M= 24, SD= 9) were considered. The sample of typical people (control group) consisted of 40 participants (24 women and 16 men). They were matched by age to the experimental group, and their age range oscillated between 17 and 40 years old (M= 20, SD= 5). IQ was not considered as an inclusion factor since pre-attentive cognitive emotional bias does not relate to intellectual capacity but peripheral information processing regulated by amygdala functioning (Adolphs & Tranel, 2004; Dolan, 2000). Reaction time measurements only relate to IQ under special experimental circumstances (Jensen, 2006). Even so, information on this matter was also recorded for information purposes.

In this follow up affective priming study, a stimulus set composed of 18 emotional faces was used. This facial set was obtained from a standardized emotional face database (BE-Face; Morales, Lopez & Hedlefs, 2010), with examples provided in Figure 3.4.

Notice from the figure that three types of emotional faces were considered: Positive, negative and neutral. These were combined through a two-way repeated measures factorial design: 3 (priming factor: Positive (P), negative (N) and neutral (Nu)) x 3 (target factor: Positive (P), negative (N) and neutral (Nu). Thus nine experimental conditions are obtained: Two emotional congruent conditions (P-P, N-N), one congruent non emotional condition that served as control (Nu-Nu); two emotional incongruent groups (P-N, N-P); and four neutral vs. emotional stimuli incongruent groups (P-Nu, N-Nu, Nu-P, Nu-N).

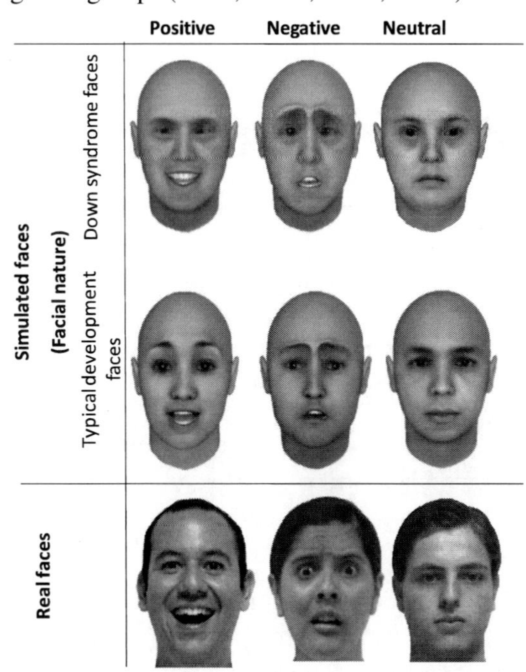

Figure 3.4. A sample of simulated and real emotional faces from a standardized facial data base (BE-Face) used in an affective priming study.

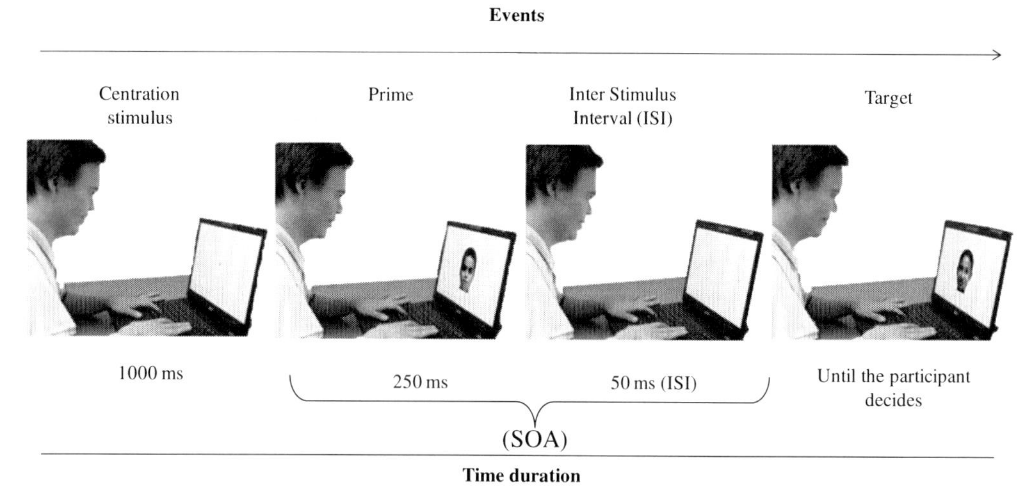

Figure 3.5. A DS participant during an affective priming experimental essay with an emotion face recognition task.

Each experimental condition represents a specific prime-target combination to be used in affective priming experimental essays. In the study, a dot appeared at the center of a computer screen to center participant's gaze. Following that, facial prime-target pairs were presented by using an ISI of 50 milliseconds and a SOA of 300 milliseconds. The experimental task was to indicate by pressing a computer keyboard key if facial targets had emotional content or not (emotion vs. no emotion) as shown in Figure 3.5.

The data analysis considered only 12 out of 20 participants with DS, as is shown in Table 3.1. This was because 8 participants never finished the study for several reasons (including dropping out, difficulties in understanding the experimental task, tiredness and death). Also, only 12 out of the 40 typical participants (TP) from the control group were considered due to practical reasons (chronological age matching, size sample equivalence, etc.).

Table 3.1. Description of personal characteristics to both study samples (Morales, 2010)

Condition	Total	Women	Men	Chronological age		Mental age	
				Mean	SD	Mean	SD
DS	12	6	6	26.08	10.98	17.49	7.48
TP	12	6	6	22.91	7.37	22.88	7.69

Results showed that not all participants with DS have difficulties in recognizing negative facial information (two out of the twelve correctly recognized all negative targets). However, since ten participants with DS failed to correctly recognize 80% or 100% of negative targets, only six experimental conditions were taken into account when applying an ANOVA statistical analysis (Table 3.2).

Table 3.2. Analysis of Variance results for the current affective priming study exploring DS emotional preference as well as emotion recognition difficulties

Source	df	F	η2	P
Group	1	19.22	.46	.0002
Error	22			
Emotional congruency	5	6.43	.22	0.00002
Group * Emotional congruency	5	1.80	.07	0.11
Error	110			

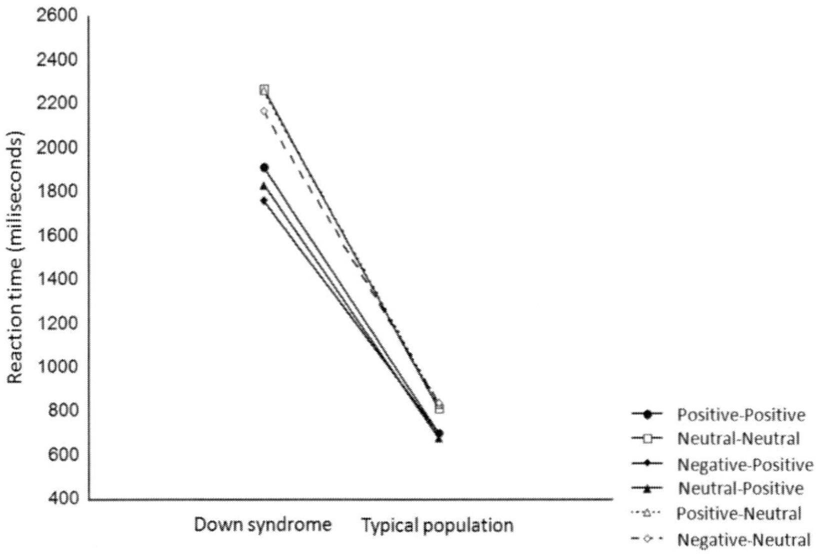

Figure 3.6. Interaction graph between the group type and emotional face pairs congruency (Morales, 2004).

Table 3.3. Post hoc comparisons for congruency and group type

Level	Comparison	Group	*df*	F	*p*
Congruent	PP-NuNu	Experimental	1	4.84	.03
		Control	1	.48	.49
		Error	22		
Incongruent	PP-NP	Experimental	1	10.07	.004
		Control	1	.002	.96
		Error	22		
	PP-NuP	Experimental	1	5.12	.03
		Control	1	.31	.57
		Error	22		
	NP-NuP	Experimental	1	2.63	.11
		Control	1	.14	.70
		Error	22		

The ANOVA results suggest a significant performance difference between groups. This difference can be attributed to the DS low cognitive factor as compared to typical ability. However, it is worth noting that whereas participants with DS only received differential priming patterns for positive and neutral, this was not the case for the control group (see Figure 3.6).

Overall, these results suggest that DS improper automatic appraisals of emotional facial information cannot be generalized to the entire population with this condition. On the other hand, recognition of positive facial information depends on previous contextual emotional information. Taking into cosideration this last observation, post hoc comparisons were carried over experimental conditions where the targets were positive. Table 3.3 shows the results of these comparisons.

As can be seen in Table 3.3, with the experimental group, the positive/positive latencies were significantly higher than neutral/neutral pair latencies. Also notice that the second comparison (positive/positive-negative/positive) contained the highest latency difference. This suggests that in contrast to the study sample with typical people, DS participants seemed to have a preference for positive information. This is particularly so whenever positive information relates to automatic processing of emotional information.

In order to look deeper into the DS emotion appraisal system, Morales and Lopez (2011) explored the question of whether a familiarity factor might regulate as it did in previous studies automatic appraisals of emotional face recognition. By using the same affective prime design with simulated familiar and non familiar emotion faces (Figure 3.4), they required DS and typical participants to perform the same emotional classification tasks. Although more ecological validity is obtained if natural faces are included, this option was not considered since DS subjects had major difficulties in emulating some emotional negative faces (Figure 3.7). Let us pause to consider this.

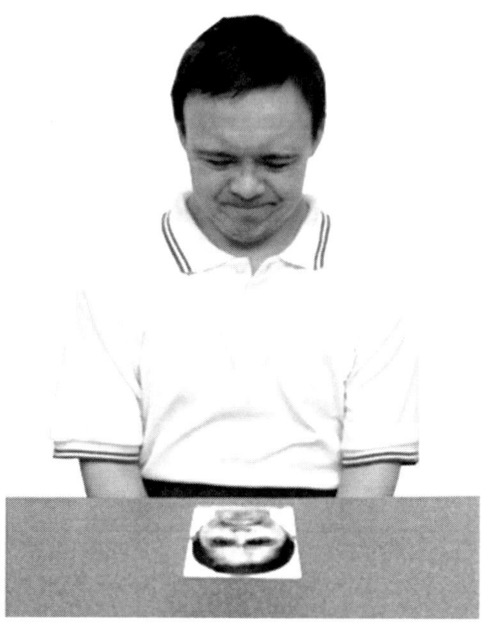

Figure 3.7. Some DS participants can not exactly imitate negative facial information (e.g. anger).

First, difficulty in voluntarily reproducing or recognizing negative faces does not necessarily imply they have an emotional deficit. As noted earlier, some study participants classified negative face photos as non emotional since these kinds of faces are not the same as positive faces, and because of this they did not like them. Consider the following comments from one of these participants:

"I told you I am a Down person, and Down people are never angry"
"I do not like to be angry"
"I am a happy person"

These remarks as well as the reviewed research up to here suggest the possibility of a DS emotional system, biased to positively perceive environmental information.

As suggested in the previous chapter, another possibility regarding the difficulty of people with DS to voluntary reproduce negative facial information is that it may be related to some self-monitoring processing aspects of their own emotional experiences. Let us consider the case of a photo session where one of the study participants with DS was unsuccessfully trying to reproduce a negative face (he was smiling instead of imitating an angry face: Figure 4.7). Here, as a performance feedback, a mirror was used to show this person that his emotional facial expression (smiling) did not correspond to a negative face (e.g. anger, fear, etc.). He and other participants denied the fact that they were smiling (self-awareness absence) and some unsuccessfully tried to modify their facial expression by using the mirror (self-monitoring limitations).

A follow up exploration on this emotional behaviour required participants with DS to identify and discriminate emotional faces from previous affective priming studies. Specifically, they were presented with a random set of faces and asked to decide which ones had emotional content. Then these faces were presented in pairs and they had to decide if both faces were emotional or if one of the faces showed no emotion (Figure 3.8). Finally, they had to name the emotion presented in each face.

Participants that had more than a 60% identification error in at least one of the required tasks, received a second explanation regarding what an emotion is, by presenting them face examples for each positive and negative emotion as well as examples of neutral faces. They were then required to go through the identifications and discrimination tasks again. If a participant failed on this second trial, the participant was classified as having some emotional limitation. If she or he succeeded, then the participants retried emotional face imitation. Even so, it was difficult to obtain a DS real emotional face set. This is why it was necessary to simulate familiar and non familiar emotional faces based on real DS neutral faces (face morphing). Figure 3.9., shows an affective priming experimental essay using these simulated emotional faces.

Again, as expected from previous research, not all participants showed DS negative face recognition deficits (Morales & Lopez, 2010). Interestingly, in contrast to the control group, no affective priming can be obtained for non familiar positive targets in the sample with DS. This was not the case for familiar positive facial information that typifies this sample as persons with DS (DS simulated emotional faces) (see Figure 3.10). This is consistent with face recognition research suggesting familiarity effects regarding the recognition of a face (Doubis, Roosin, Schiltz, Boardt, Crommelinck, 1999; Lund, 2001; Parkin, 1999)

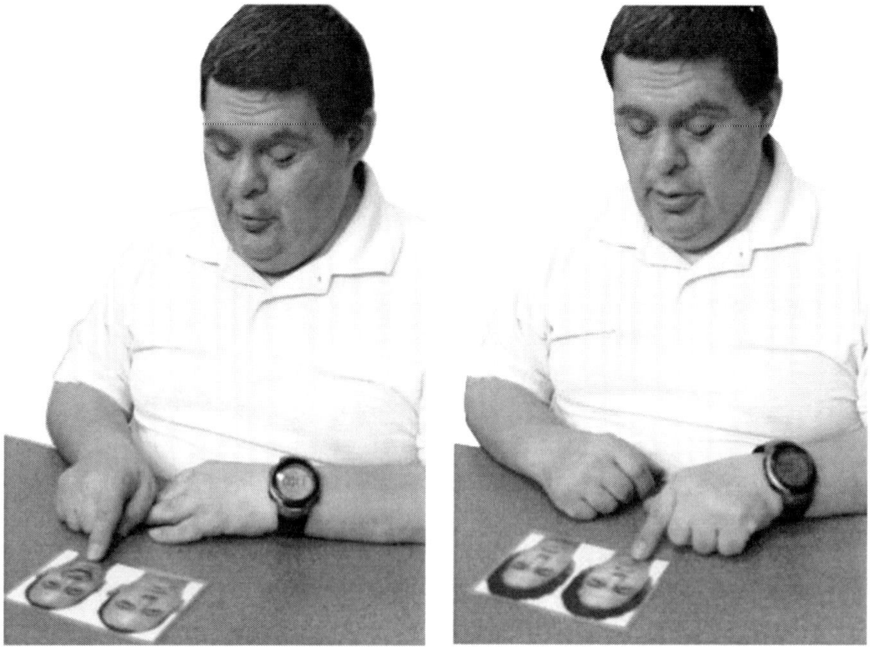

Figure 3.8. An emotional discrimination task. Here, a DS participant had to point: a) The face showing a positive feeling (left panel), b) the face showing a negative feeling (right panel).

Overall, the above affective priming studies suggest that people with DS have a strong bias toward processing positive information, and they are more sensitive than typical individuals to familiar face information, especially if these positive faces are familiar.

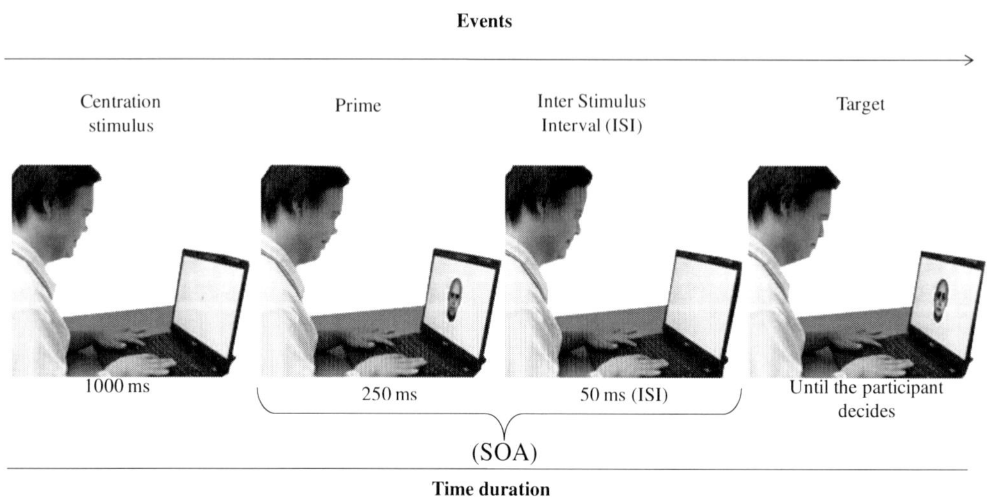

Figure 3.9. A DS participant taking an affective priming experimental essay.

Let us conclude remarks on the affective priming paradigm by saying that it can be used in many other ways to study people with DS's perception of facial information. For example, in order to explore emotion face recognition mechanisms in this population another affective priming study was carried over to determine if perceiving an emotional face (Familiar or non familiar) obeys analytical or configurational face cognitive processing. This research was done using stimuli inversion (upward and downward oriented faces).

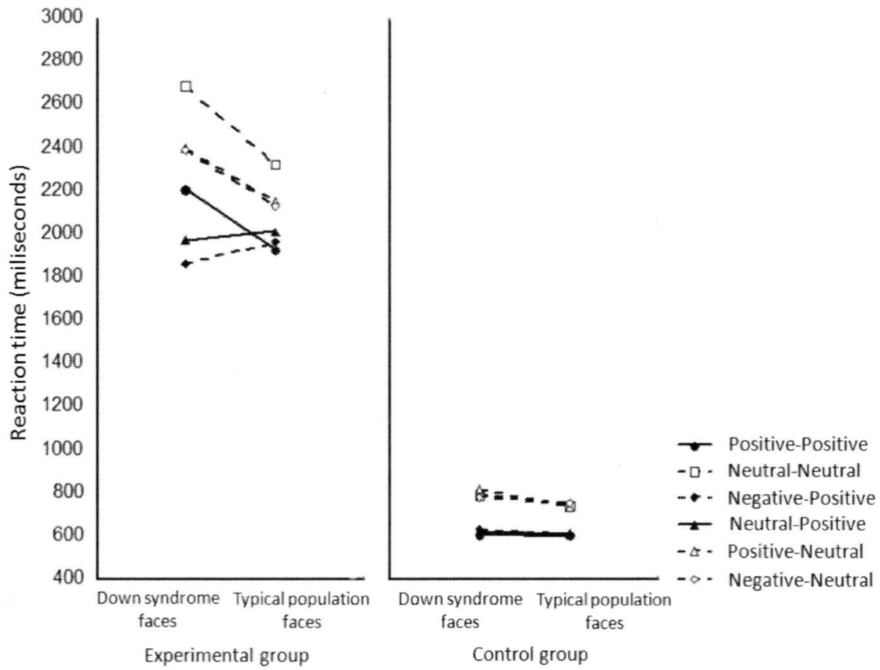

Figure 3.10. Interaction pattern for group type, familiarity and emotional congruency (Morales, 2010).

Research using recognition of downward rotated faces has been used to determine the specific visual mechanisms involved in face recognition. In DS visual research, some visual inversion research has been conducted to analyze how members of this population visually process specific facial components. For instance, Wishart and Pitcairn (2000) explored in this population identity and facial expression recognition (familiar and non familiar) using face inversion. Here, they required children to choose a face they have seen previously among a group. Again, children with DS were slower and committed more mistakes than typical children (matched by chronological age). Additional visual research supports these results (e.g., Annaz et al., 2009). In particular, Wang, Doherty, Rourke and Bellugi (1995), reported that people with DS tested with lower recognition scores in the Benton test than people with the same age having Williams syndrome (WS). Moreover, in the aforementioned study from Wishart and Pitcairn, in contrast to typical participants, people with DS showed insensitivity to face rotation (Williams et al., 2005; Wishart, et al., 2007). Due to the absence of a face rotation effect it has been suggested that the DS's visual face recognition system must be mainly based on analytical processing (Annaz et al., 2009).

Considering that this visual research mainly relied on results from very young participants, the possibility arises that the way of analyzing facial information may change with maturity. This is worth considering since some visual research suggests significant differences in scores between young and adult subjects' face information processing (Schwarzer, 2000). On this matter, Morales and Lopez have recently conducted an affective priming study to look for age differences in face information processing. The test was designed to see if the DS perceptual system might be differently tuned to process specific components aspects of a face (analytical processing) depending on the age, or if they process face components based on their spatial relation (configuration processing). Thus in the affective priming study some emotional face primes were inverted (see Figure 3.11). The study expected to find that since visual inversion tends to diminish face configuration processing (Prkachin, 2003; Valentine, 1988) then no affective priming should be obtained for inverted primes.

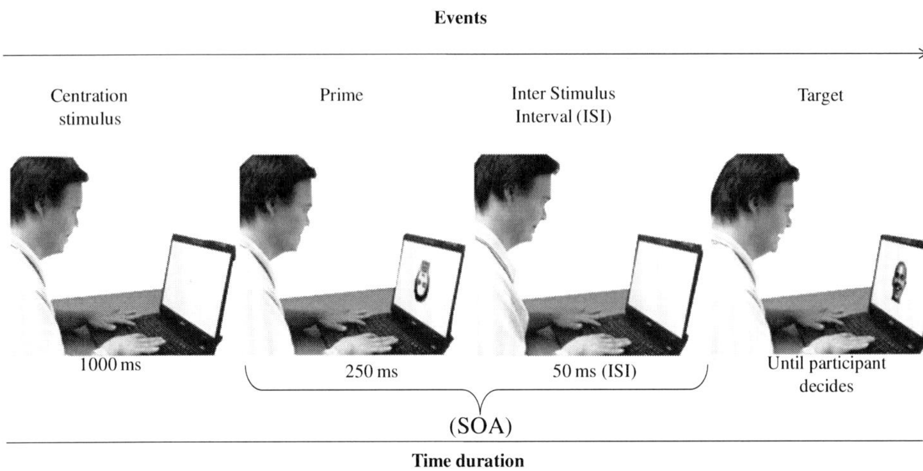

Figure 3.11. A DS participant going through an affective experimental essay with an inverted face prime.

In this inverted emotional faces study, ten out of twelve participants with DS displayed difficulties in recognizing negative facial information. For this reason, data analysis only considered experimental condition comparisons where the target was positive (see Table 3.4).

Table 3.4. Comparisons between emotional congruency and face rotation for each group

Comparison Upward face vs. Downward face	Group	*Df*	F	*p*
Positive/Positive	Experimental	1	1.05	.31
	Control	1	.10	.75
	Error	22		
Negative/Positive	Experimental	1	5.48	.02
	Control	1	.03	.84
	Error	22		
Neutral/Positive	Experimental	1	4.42	.04
	Control	1	.02	.88
	Error	22		
Neutral/Neutral	Experimental	1	1.57	.22
	Control	1	.01	.90
	Error	22		

The results from Table 3.4, as well as those shown in the interaction graphs from Figure 3.12., seem to suggest that participants with DS possess a face configuration processing style when positive information is considered. This can be observed from the P-P experimental condition where the inverted face prime destroys the affective prime over the target. It is not clear if this is also the case for negative face information where an upward negative face has no facilitation or interference on recognizing a positive target. However, a downward negative face affects the recognition of a positive face by significantly increasing the response latency.

One clear implication from these last findings is the possibility that negative information can be implicitly processed even before it can be recognized. This is suggested by previous negative face information context influence recognition of positive facial information. This can also be identified throughout the three previous studies, in which participants with DS consciously showed difficulties in recognizing negative information. This peculiar emotional behaviour leads to the hypothesis that perhaps some very low perceptual mechanisms (peripheral processing) might be involved, even before the start of controlled/conscious attentive processes.

In the spirit of providing another cognitive methodology with which to deal with this kind of emotional behaviour, let us briefly illustrate how computer simulations can be used to explore this hypothesis of peripheral cognitive processing of emotional face recognition on populations with DS.

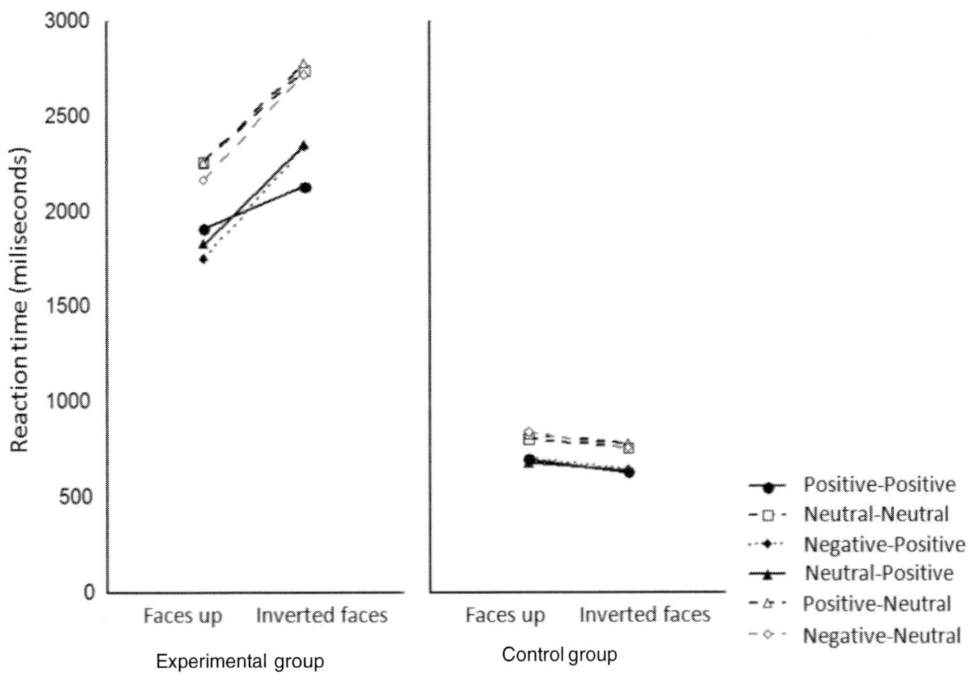

Figure 3.12. Interaction graph for Group * Facial orientation * Emotional congruency.

3.3.3. Down Syndrome and Facial Emotion Perception from a Neuro-Computational Perspective

In the early days of cognitive psychology, mental activity was genrally described using a computer metaphor. In the middle of heated theoretical debates, this approach introduced a new interdisciplinary paradigm to explore mental life from another academic perspective, thus the cognitive Human Information Processing approach was born in the early twenty century (HIP). At first, it was not common practice to include the brain physiology underlying cognitive functioning, and sometimes this explanation level was avoided. At present, especially among young cognitive scientists, using different explanation levels to explore our mind is more acceptable in discussing cognitive theory development (mathematical, computational, physiological, and psychological). It is now more common to model cognitive behaviour from a connectionist point of view. Specifically, the connectionist approach to explain mental fucntions assumes that studying our brain's computational properties through biologically-inspired computation machines (which use simulated synaptic connectivity of simulated neuron units) makes it possible to test cognitive hypothesis about our brains' physiology (Churchland (a), 1986; Churchland (b), 1996, 2007; Hougton, 2005; Rogers & McClelland, 2004) under academic scrutiny.

Let us keep in mind that people with DS have difficulties in recognizing negative facial information and have an explicit preference and automatic processing bias to positive information. Also, there is a chance that this particular way of processing emotional information is related to some specific peripheral low-level perceptual mechanism(s), rather than a high-level conceptual mechanism. Since peripheral face recognition mechanisms are neurocomputational-oriented, a connectionist approach would appear to be suitable for studying this DS negative-positive recognition hypothesis. Morales and Lopez documented some research on this topic (Morales & Lopez, 2012). However before we can describe this connectionist research it will be necessary a brief introduction to cognitive face recognition theory.

Face recognition research is a fascinating area, that has been approached from many points of view (for a review, see Delac, & Grgic, 2007; Valentine, 1995). As humans, we are capable from very early in life (a few minutes after we are born Acerra, Burnod, & Schonen, 2002; Johnstons & Ellis, 1995; Schwarzer, Zauner & Korell, 2003) of recognizing facial information in a rudimentary way. This innate visual capacity has brought academic attention to study a wide set of face recognition variables like stimulus contrast, brightness, color, etc. or spatial relation or configuration aspects of face components (Morton & Johnson, 1991; Mondloch, Lewis, Budreau, Maurer, Dannemiller, Stephens & Kleiner-Gathercoal, 1999; Schwarzer et al., 2003; Zebrowitz, 2006) using a wide variety of research methods and techniques such as remembering facial information (Pine, Lissek, Klein, Mannuzza, Moulton, Guardino & Woldehawariat, 2004; Reynolds & Pezdek, 1992), brain neuro imaging analysis (Herba & Phillips, 2004), face recognition tests (Christensen, Riley, Heffernan, Love & MacLaughlin Sta.Maria, 2002), etc. However, at the risk of being overly simplistic, it is worth to our current chapter section to confine our theoretical arguments on face recognition to a cognitive modelling approach.

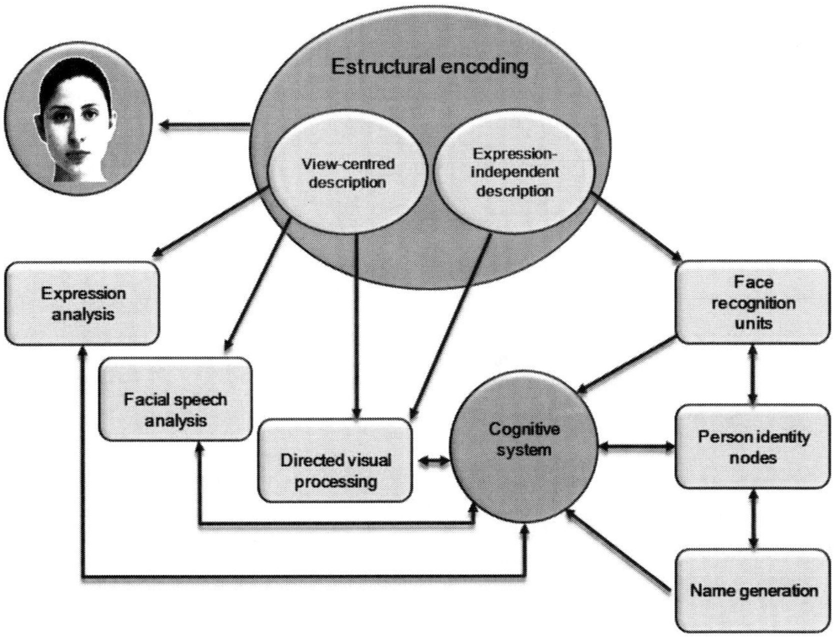

Figure 3.13. A top down face recognition chart, where incoming face information (structural encoding of several types of information) is recognized and identified as belonging to someone, and activating a proper name to the identified person.

One of the most seminal and representative cognitive models of face recognition was introduced by Bruce and Young in 1986. In this sequential processing model, it is assumed that facial information is firstly encoded structurally if the information matches an existing Face Recognition Unit (FRU). This will in turn be activated, as well as any related physical information and semantic knowledge. This then activates a related Person Identity Node (PIN), which accesses personal information, such as occupation, interests, etc. Finally, a name for the identified person is generated. According to this model, names are stored separately from the FRUs and PIN units, but can only be accessed via the PIN (see Figure 3.13).

In this face recognition model, familiar and unfamiliar faces are processed in different ways. For instance, unfamiliar faces cannot use FRUs, PIN units or name generation. Familiar and unfamiliar faces activate expression analysis, speech analysis, or directed visual processing.

Criticism to this model includes observations about non specificity regarding how FRUs and PIN units develop, and how emotional processing specifically participates on face recognition (e.g., Lund, 2001). Furthermore, the assumption of holistic or configuration processing in this model has also been challenged, since there is evidence that specific face components are extremely relevant to face recognition (eyes, mouth, etc.; Collishaw & Hole, 2000).

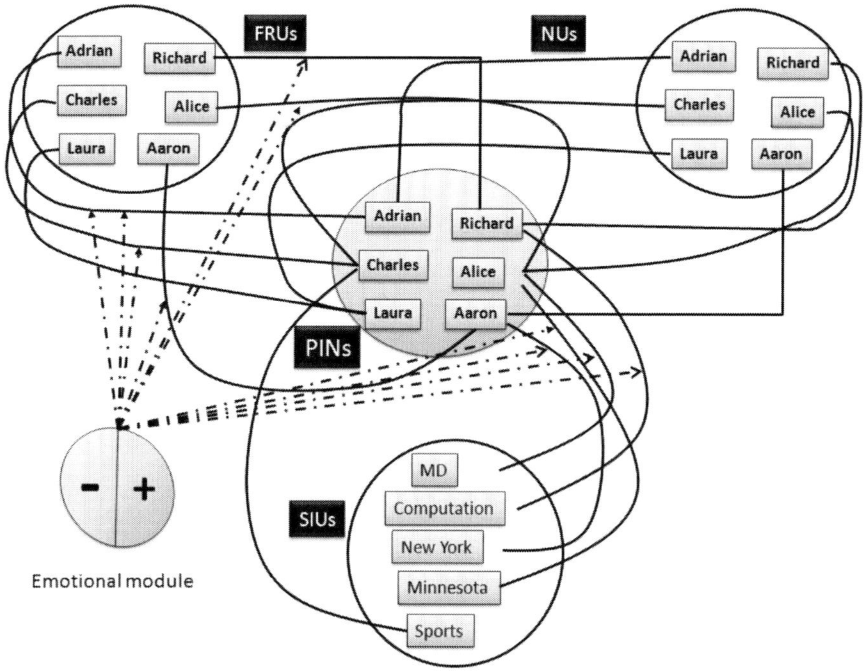

Figure 3.14. An alternative face recognition model where a simulated amygdala has an effect over a classic model of human face recognition composed of Face Recognition Units (FRUs), Person Identity Nodes (PINs), Semantic Information Units (SIUs) and Name Units (NUs).

Modern alternative cognitive face recognition models have some trouble coping with Bruce and Young's model limitations. For instance, more specificity is demanded regarding emotion mechanisms participating in the face recognition process (Herzmann, Schweinberger, Sommer & Jentzsch, 2004). Accordingly, Breen et al. (2000) presented a connectionist face recognition model that addresses emotional face information. Specifically, this model acknowledges two routes by which facial information is processed. One route relates to recognition of face identity (like in Bruce and Young's model), and the other route (non conscious/automatic) is to process emotional face information. This hypothetical model finds some support from both familiar and non familiar face recognition research (Bobes, Lopera, Coma, Galan, Carbonell, Bringas & Valdes-Sosa, 2004; Quinones, Pérez, Leon & Bobes, 2006).

The Breen et al.' s face recognition model can be used to explore the hypothesis that DS negative face recognition limitations are related to peripheral low-level perception mechanisms. Specifically, a computer simulation of a connectionist (dual model) face recognition model can be built where a simulated amygdala is specifically used to affect recognition of facial information as is illustrated in Figure 3.14.

Here, the simulated amygdala provides emotional face information during the face recognition process. This emotional information is not related to stored emotional content as in Bruce and Young's model, but to recognition of emotional valence of face stimuli through an alternative processing rout as suggested by Breen et al.' s model. Damage to this simulated emotional system might bring insightful ideas about DS emotional system as it is discussed next.

Testing properties of the human visual system through computer simulation allows us to check (among other things) if the hypothesis about visual perception has computational plausibility. This is the case for connectionist computer simulations used to test if specific neural computation may underlie visual behaviour. Then, if peripheral visual processing is related to DS negative recognition deficits then at least some neural computation plausibility to this assumption must be probed.

In order to explore whether constrained amygdala circuitry may affect very low visual mechanisms underlying face recognition in a specific way, a set of connectionist computer simulations were implemented by Morales & Lopez (2012). The general idea was to build a neural net to emulate simple amygdala computation in interacting and regulating emotional facial information based on some Breen et al.'s model guidelines (2000). The general idea is presented in Figure 3.15.

In the study a 64 retina units wide x 48 units high (3072 units) size worked as visual stimuli receptors. In turn, this retina fed forwarded input into a hidden kohonen neural layer composed of 60 units, that in turn passed information to a 14 unit identity recognition layer (one unit for each face to recognize), where each unit competes to identify an incoming face (Interactive Activation Competition system; Rumelhart,1986).

First, the simulated amygdala was trained to discriminate positive, negative and neutral faces. There were two amygdala systems, one for DS face recognition and another one specialized to recognize typical population faces. This was done by presenting to the retina the Eigenface (obtained by principal component analysis: PCA) for each emotional face. This assures better neural net recognition performance. PCA converts the pixels of an image into a number of Eigenface feature vectors, which provides salient information from a face (for a complete mathematical description of this process see Eleyan & Demirel, 2007). Figure 3.16. shows some examples of using PCA to obtain Eigenfaces.

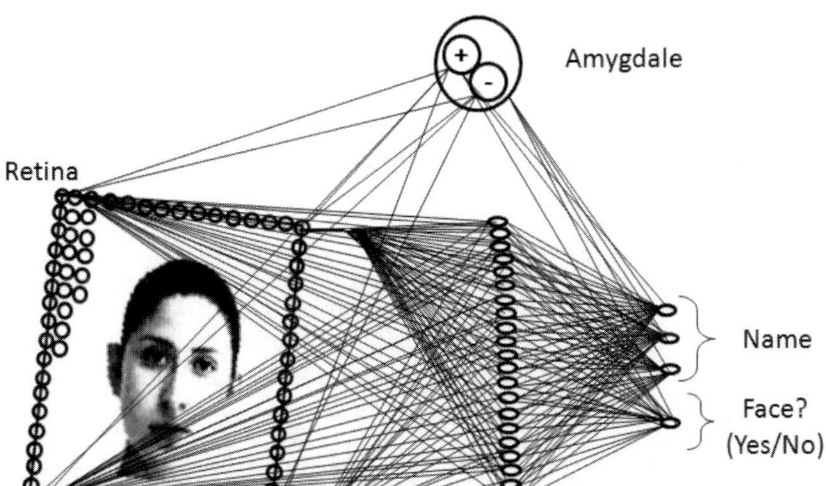

Figure 3.15. A neural net architecture. After training the simulated amygdala functioning, it is damaged to test for negative face recognition deficits.

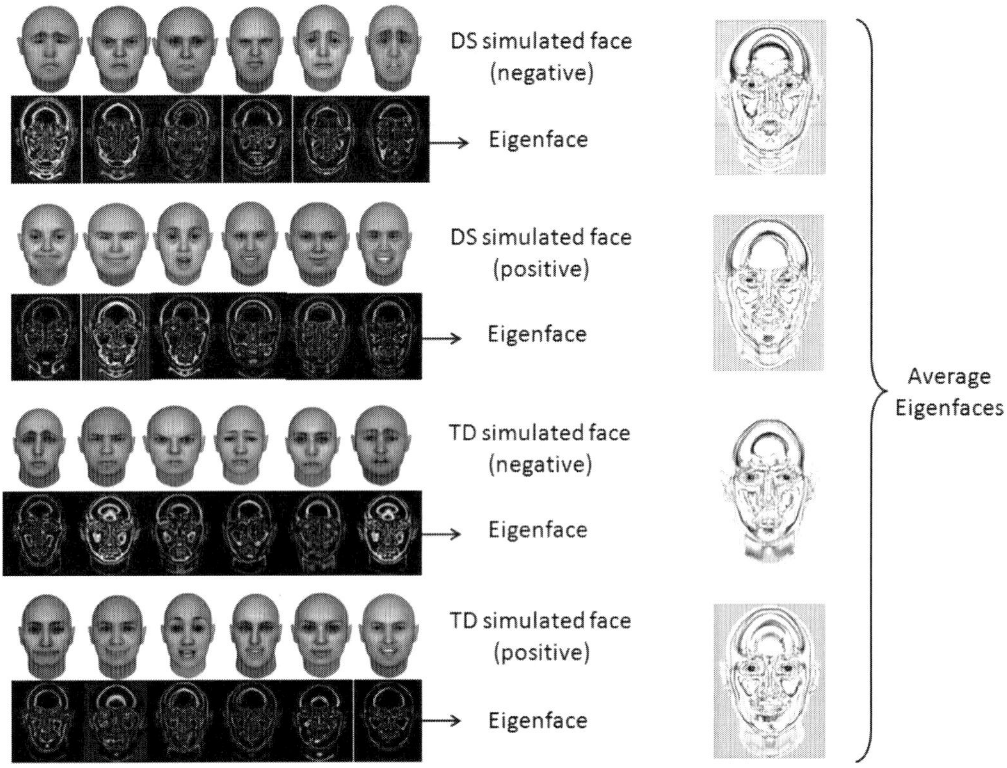

Figure 3.16. Examples of Eigenfaces (in black) for DS and TD emotional faces used to train a neural net. The average Eigenface for each set is presented.

Table 3.5 shows the neural net's performance after unsupervised learning of both populations' emotional faces. Notice from the table that no perfect discrimination was obtained. Rather, each neuron converged to discriminate between positive and negative faces. However, negative face recognition can be obtained using this simple architecture. That is, there is some computational plausibility to the idea that we sustain early visual discriminatory processing of emotional faces using only implicit facial information.

As can be seen from Table 3.6, better performance is obtained if a backward backpropagation error is provided to the neural net, to adjust "synaptic connectivity" during recognition training (to perfect classification for negative faces).

The fact that positive faces could not be grouped into a single face classification might be due to the possibility that some of these faces share more facial negative facial characteristics than other positive faces and thus they are misclassified as negative faces. Take for instance the third DS positive face stimulus from Table 3.6 (a surprise face), that was classified as positive. This is incorrect: neuron 1 is supposed to respond only to negative information. Howver, this is possible since a facial expression of surprise shares many facial characteristics with a fear face (see Figure 3.17).

Modifications to the neural architecture (e.g. including or deleting competitive neurons) and changing learning paradigms did not improve face recognition performance. If only one neural net is trained to recognize both population faces, then face recognition decreases (see Table 3.8). Facial characteristics from both population face sets caused interference in the convergence into proper face recognition. Neural net modifications did not improve face recognition performance.

Table 3.5. After intensive training, both amygdala neurons (1 or 2) showed some identification to Positive Faces stimuli (PF; 1-6) or Negative Faces Stimuli (NF; 7-12) with DS and TD emotional Eigenfaces

UNSUPERVISED LEARNING

TYPICAL DEVELOPMENT FACES (TD)					DOWN SYNDROME FACES (DS)				
Neuron	1		2			1		2	
	Response to negative	Response to positive	Response to negative	Response to positive		Response to negative	Response to positive	Response to negative	Response to positive
Faces									
PF. 1				•	PF. 1				•
PF. 2		•			PF. 2				•
PF. 3		•			PF. 3				•
PF. 4				•	PF. 4				•
PF. 5		•			PF. 5		•		
PF. 6				•	PF. 6		•		
NF. 1	•				NF. 1			•	
NF. 2	•				NF. 2			•	
NF. 3	•				NF. 3			•	
NF. 4	•				NF. 4	•			
NF. 5	•				NF. 5	•			
NF. 6	•				NF. 6	•			

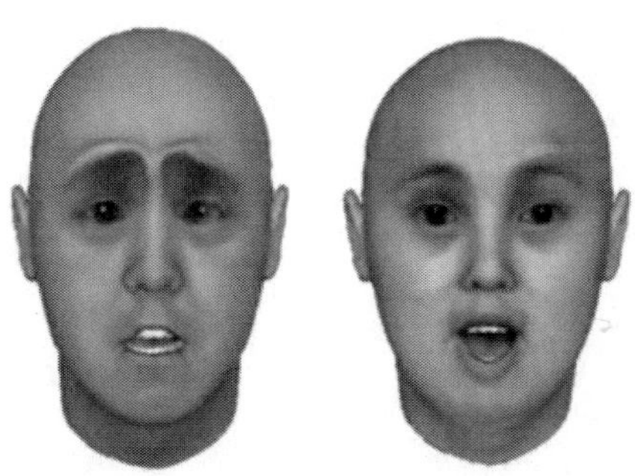

Figure 3.7. A fear face (left) and a surprise face (right) are mistakenly classified due to possible facial similarities.

Table 3.6. Backpropagation Neural net's performance in emotional face recognition

SUPERVISED LEARNING

TYPICAL DEVELOPMENT FACES (TD)					DOWN SYNDROME FACES (DS)				
Neuron	1		2			1		2	
	Response to negative	Response to positive	Response to negative	Response to positive		Response to negative	Response to positive	Response to negative	Response to positive
Faces									
PF. 1				•	PF. 1				•
PF. 2		•			PF. 2				•
PF. 3		•			PF. 3		•		
PF. 4				•	PF. 4				•
PF. 5		•			PF. 5				•
PF. 6				•	PF. 6				•
NF. 1	•				NF. 1	•			
NF. 2	•				NF. 2	•			
NF. 3	•				NF. 3	•			
NF. 4	•				NF. 4	•			
NF. 5	•				NF. 5	•			
NF. 6	•				NF. 6	•			

In order to test the entire emotional face recognition system, only the group of faces that were correctly classified in the previous simulation were used to train the new amygdala system (three positive, three negative, and three neutral faces). The FRU units as well as PIN units (see Figure 3.14.) promptly converged toward a global minimum error in correctly recognizing all neutral and emotional facial faces. After this, amygdala dysfunction was induced to emulate DS negative face recognition deficits.

Damage to amygdala was simulated by introducing connectivity noise between the retina and the amygdala. Interestingly enough, only the negative face recognition—in almost its entirety—was affected. The recognition of positive faces as well as the normal functioning of FRU and PIN units was unaffected. Another consideration of damage to amygdala (like connectivity damage) is that it always brought deficits first in recognizing negative information, and only after considerable more damage, affected other neural nets' recognition capacities.

All in all, this kind of academic exploration suggests that emotional facial information possesses explicit and implicit information that can be detected by low-level perception mechanisms. By constraining neural computations underlying emotion information processing (like the genetically constrained DS's emotional system), the most strongly affected information emotion recognition capacity relates to negative information. More visual perception research is in demand to determine how much of DS negative recognition functioning is based on peripheral processing rather than conceptual.

Table 3.8. The amygdala's face classification results to both populations' emotional faces

SUPERVISED LEARNING (ALL)

TYPICAL DEVELOPMENT FACES (TD)					DOWN SYNDROME FACES (DS)				
Neuron	1		2			1		2	
	Response to negative	Response to positive	Response to negative	Response to positive		Response to negative	Response to positive	Response to negative	Response to positive
Faces									
PF. 1		•			PF. 1				•
PF. 2		•			PF. 2		•		
PF. 3		•			PF. 3		•		
PF. 4		•			PF. 4				•
PF. 5				•	PF. 5		•		
PF. 6		•			PF. 6				•
NF. 1	•				NF. 1			•	
NF. 2	•				NF. 2			•	
NF. 3	•				NF. 3			•	
NF. 4	•				NF. 4			•	
NF. 5	•				NF. 5			•	
NF. 6	•				NF. 6			•	

3.4. Final Words

To review, the above academic research outlines a profound message about the emotional world of people with DS. They use a different crystal to emotionalize the world where we all live. In fact, this chapter leads to a suggestion of the prevalence of an emotional affective style that typifies them as a particular group among us. Salient characteristics of this emotional style are: a) A non typical high preference for positive emotion, b) an emotional system for processing negative information that behaves in different ways depending on instances of controlled or automatic cognitive processing, and c) a configuration style mode of processing facial information. With the above research, we have introduced some types of cognitive methods of exploring emotions and DS. This exploration is guided on the belief that not all people with DS can be classified as "having an emotional deficit". Instead, emotional variability inside this population suggests a genetic constrained emotional style leading to a particular way of experiencing emotion. As we will review in the next following chapters, this emotional style has strong implication about how members of this population signify a wide behaviour range, including moral behaviour, love, happiness, etc.

References

Acerra, F., Burnod, Y. & Schonen, S. (2002). Modelling aspects of face processing in early infancy. *Developmental Science*, *5*(1), 98-117. doi: 10.1111/1467-7687.00215

Adolphs, R. & Tranel, D. (2004). Impaired judgments of sadness but not happiness following bilateral amygdala damage. *Journal of Cognitive Neuroscience*, *16*(3), 453–462.

Adolphs, R., Tranel, D. & Damasio, A. R. (1998). The human amygdala in social judgment. *Nature*, *393*, 460-474. doi: 10.1038/30982

Annaz, D., Karmiloff-Smith, A., Johnson, M. H. & Thomas, M. S. C. (2009). A cross-syndrome study of the development of holistic face recognition in children with autism, Down syndrome, and Williams syndrome. *Journal of Experimental Child Psychology*, *102*(4), 456-486. Retrieved from http://www.psyc.bbk.ac.uk/research/DNL/personalpages /annaz_etal_2009.pdf

Bargh, J. A. (1999). The cognitive monster: the case against the controllability of automatic stereotype effects. In S. Chaiken & Y. Trope (Eds.). *Dual process theories in social psychology* (pp. 361-382). New York, NY, EE. UU.: Guilford Press.

Benda, C. E. (1971). Mongolism. In J. Minckler (Ed.). *Pathology of the nervous system* (pp. 1361-1371). New York, NY, EE. UU.: McGraw-Hill.

Blair, R. J. R., Morris, J. S., Frith, C. D., Perrett, D. I., & Dolan, R. J. (1999). Dissociable neural responses to facial expressions of sadness and anger. *Brain, 122*, 883-893.

Bobes, M. A., Lopera, F., Coma, L. D., Galan, L., Carbonell, F., Bringas, M. L. & Valdés-Sosa, M. (2004). Brain potentials reflect residual face processing in a case of prosopagnosia. *Cognitive Neuropsychology, 21*(7), 691-718. Retrieved from http://www.ece.uvic.ca/~bctill/papers/facerec/Bobes_etal_2004.pdf

Breen, N., Caine, D. & Coltheart, M. (2000). Models of face recognition and delusional misidentification: a critical review. *Cognitive Neuropsychology, 17*(1-3), 55-71.

Bruce, V. & Young, A. (1986). Understanding face recognition. *British Journal of Psychology, 77*(3), 305-327. doi: 10.1111/j.2044-8295.1986.tb02199.x

Calder, A. (2003). The perception of Facial Expressions. *Cognition and Brain Sciences Unit.* Retrieved May 12, 2003 from, http://www.mrccbu.cam.ac.uk/personal/andy.calder/ perception.shtml

Carvajal, F. & Iglesias, J. (2002). Face-to-face emotion interaction studies in Down syndrome infants. *International Journal of Behavioural Development*, *26*(2), 104-112. doi: 10.1080/01650250042000609

Christensen, K. J., Riley, B. E., Heffernan, K. A., Love, S. B. & McLaughlin Sta. Maria, M. E. (2002). Facial recognition test in the elderly: norms, reliability and premorbid estimation. *Clinical Neuropsychology 16*(1): 51-6. doi: 10.1076/clin.16.1.51.8332

Chung, M. S. & Donald, M. T. (1995). Development of face recognition. *The British Journal of Psychology, 86*, 55-87.

Churchland, P. S. (1986). *Neurophilosophy: Towars a unified science of the Mind/Brain.* Nueva York, NY, EE. UU.: Bradford Book.

Churchland, P. M. (2007). *Neurophilosophy at work.* Cambridge: Cambridge University Press.

Churchland, P. M. (1996). *The engine of reason, the seat of the soul: A philosophical journey into the brain.* Cambridge, Massachusetts: The MIT Press.

Collishaw, S. M., & Hole, G. J. (2000). Featural and configurational processes in the recognition of faces of different familiarity. *Perception, 29*, 893–909. doi: 10.1068/p2949

Conrad, N. J., Schmidt, L. A., Niccols, A., Polak, C. P., Riniolo, T. C. & Burack, J. A. (2007). Frontal electroencephalogram asymmetry during affective processing in children with Down syndrome: a pilot study. *Journal of Intellectual Disability Research, 51*(12), 988-995. doi: 10.1111/j.1365-2788.2007.01010.x. ISSN: 0964-2633.

Davidson, R. J. (2003). Affective neuroscience and psychophysiology: Toward a synthesis. Psychophysiology, 40, 655-665.

Davidson, R. J. (2004). Well-being and affective style: Neural substrates and biobehavioural correlates. *Philosophical Transactions of the Royal Society (London), 359*, 1395-1411. doi: 10.1098/rstb.2004.1510

Davidson, R. J. (1998). Affective style and affective disorders: Perspectives from affective neuroscience. *Cognition and Emotion, 12(3)*, 307-320. Retrieved from http://psyphz.psych.wisc.edu/web/pubs/1998/Affective_style.pdf

Davidson, R. J., Putnam, K. M. & Larson, C. L. (2000). Dysfunction in the neural circuitry of emotion regulation-A possible prelude to violence. *Science, 289* 591-594. doi: 10.1126/science.289.5479.591

Davidson, R. J. & Irwin, W. (1999). The functional neuroanatomy of emotion and affective style. *Trends in cognitive sciences*, 3, 11 - 21.

De Houwer, J., Hermans, D. & Eelen, P. (1998). Affectivity and identity priming with episodically associated stimuli. *Cognition and Emotion*, *12*(2), 145-169. Retrieved from http://psyserv06.psy.sbg.ac.at:5916/fetch/PDF/15111229.pdf

Delac, K., & Grgic, M. (Eds.) (2007). *Face recognition*. Austria, Vienna: I-Tech Education and Publishing.

Dimberg, U., Thunberg, M. & Elmehed, K. (2000). Unconscious facial reactions to emotional facial expression. *Psychology Science, 11*(1), 86-89. Retrieved from http://apsychoserver.psych.arizona.edu/jjbareprints/psyc501a/readings/Dimberg_Thunberg_Elmehed_2000_Psych_Science.pdf

Dubois, S., Rossion, B., Schiltz, C., Bodart, J. M., Michel, C., Bruyer, R. & Crommelinck, M. (1999). Effect of familiarity on the processing of human faces. *NeuroImage, 9*(3), 278-289.

Dolan, R.J. (2000) Functional neuroimaging of the human amygdala during emotional processing and learning. In The Amygdala: A Functional Analysis (2nd edn) (Aggleton, J.P., ed.), pp. 631–653, Oxford University Press

Ekman, P. (2003). *Emotions reveled: recognizing faces and feelings to improve communication and emotional life*. EE. UU.: Times books.

Ekman, P., Friesen, W. V. & Hager, J. C. (2002). *Facial action coding system: the manual*. EE. UU.: Research Nexus division of Network Information Research Corporation.

Eleyan, A., y Demirel, H. (2007). PCA and LDA based Neural Networks for Human Face Recognition. In D. K. Delac & M. Grgic (Eds.). *Face Recognition* (pp. 93-106). Viena, Austria: I-TECH Education and Publishing.

Fazio, R. H. (1995). Attitudes as object-evaluation associations: Determinants, consequences, and correlates of attitude accessibility. In R. E. Petty & J. A. Krosnick (Eds.). *Attitude strength: Antecedents and consequences* (pp. 247–282). Hillsdale, NJ, EE. UU.: Erlbaum.

Fazio, R. H., Sanbonmatsu, D. M., Powell, M. C. & Kardes, F. R. (1986). On the automatic activation of attitudes. *Journal of Personality and Social Psychology, 50*(2), 229-238. doi: 10.1037/0022-3514.50.2.229

Fiedler, K. (2003). The Hidden vicissitudes of the priming paradigm in evaluative research. In J. Musch & K. C. Klauer (Eds.). *The psychology of evaluation: Affective processes in cognition and emotion* (pp. 109-137). Mahthaw, NJ., EE. UU.: LEA.

Giner-Sorolla, R., Garcia, M. T. & Bargh, J. A. (1999). The automatic evaluation of pictures. *Social Cognition, 17*(1), 76-96. doi: 10.1521/soco.1999.17.1.76

Gutiérrez, M. (2006). Procesamiento parafovial de información emocional. En E. Gámez & J. M. Díaz (Eds.). *Investigaciones en Psicología Básica ULL: Psicolingüística, Razonamiento y Emoción* (pp. 167 – 184). España: Universidad de la Laguna.

Hamann, S., & Canli, T. (2004). Individual differences in emotion processing. *Current Opinion in Neurobiology, 14*, 233–238. Doi: 10.1016/j.conb.2004.03.010

Harwood, N. K., Hall, L.J. & Schinkfield, A. J. (1999). Recognition of facial emotional expressions from moving and static displays by individuals with mental retardation. *American Journal on mental retardation, 104* (3), 270-278. Retrieved from http://www.aaiddjournals.org/doi/abs/10.1352/0895-8017(1999)104%3C0270:ROFEEF%3E2.0.CO;2

Hayes, S. C., Luoma, J., Bond, F., Masuda, A. & Lillis, J. (2006). Acceptance and commitment therapy: model, processes, and outcomes. *Behaviour Research and Therapy, 44*, 1–25. doi: 10.1016/j.brat.2005.06.006

Herba, C., & Phillips, M. (2004). Annotation: Development of facial expression recognition from childhood to adolescence: behavioural and neurological perspectives. *Journal of Child Psychology and Psychiatry, 45*(7), 1185-1198. doi: 10.1111/j.1469-7610.2004.00316.x

Hermans, D., Baeyens, F. & Eelen, P. (1998). Odours as affective-processing context for word evaluation: A case of cross- modal affective priming. *Cognition and Emotion, 12*(4), 601-613. doi: 10.1080/026999398379583

Herzmann, G., Schweinberger, S. R., Sommer, W. & Jentzsch, I. (2004). What's special about personally familiar faces? A multimodal approach. *Psychophysiology, 41*(5), 688–701. doi: 10.1111/j.1469-8986.2004.00196.x

Hofmann, S. G. & Kashdan, T. B. (2010). The affective style questionnaire: Development and psychometric properties. *J Psychopathol Behav Assess, 32,* 255–263. doi: 10.1 007/s10862-009-9142-4

Jackowski1, A. P., Laureano1, M. R., Del'Aquilla1, M. A., de Moura1, L. M., Assunção1, I., Silva1, I. & Schwartzman, J. S. (2011). Update on Clinical Features and Brain Abnormalities in Neurogenetics Syndromes. *Journal of Applied Research in Intellectual Disabilities, 24*(3), 217–236. doi: 10.1111/j.1468-3148.2010.00603.x

Jeringan, T. L., Bellugi, U., Sowell, E., Doherty, S. & Hesselink, J. R. (1993). Cerebral morphological distinctions between William's and Down's syndromes. *Archives of Neurology, 50*(2), 186-191. Retrieved from http://lcn.salk.edu/publications/1993/ Jernigan%20-%20Cerebral%20Morphologic%20Distinctions%201993.pdf

Johnstons, R.A. & Ellis, H. (1995). The development of face recognition. In: Tim Valentine. Cognitive and computational aspects of face recognition. New York: Routledge.

Kaiser, S. & Wehrle, T. (2001). *The role of facial expression in intra-individual and inter-individual emotional regulation*. Retrieved from http://www.unige.ch/faapse/emotion/members/jaiser_publ.htm.

Kelly, D. J., Quinn, P. C., Slater, A. M., Lee, K., Gibson, A., Smith, M. & Pascalis, O. (2005). Three-month-olds, but not newborns, prefer own-race faces. *Development science, 8* (6), 31-36. doi: 10.1111/j.1467-7687.2005.0434a.x

Lazarus, R. S. (2000). The cognition-emotion debate: A bit of history. In T. Dalgleish & M. Power (Eds.). *Handbook of cognition and emotion* (pp. 3-19). New York, NY, EE.UU.: John Wiley & Sons.

Lazarus, R. S. (2001). Relational meaning and discrete emotions. En K. R. Scherer, A. Schorr & T. Johnstone (Eds.). *Appraisal processes in emotion: Theory, methods, research* (pp. 3-19). Nueva York, NY, EE. UU.: Oxford University Press.

Lesch, K. P., Bengel, D., Heils, A., Sabol, S. Z., Greenberg, B. D., Petri, S. & Murphy, D. L. (1996). *Association of anxiety-related traits with a polymorphism in the serotonin transporter gene regulatory region. Science, 274*:1527-1531. Retrieved from http://www-psych.stanford.edu/~knutson/per/lesch96.pdf

Lind J., Vuorenkoski V., Rosberg G., Paratanen T. J. & Wasz-Hockert, O. (1970). Spectrographic analysis of vocal response to pain stimuli in infants with Down's syndrome. *Dev Med Child Neurol, 12*: 478–86.

Morales, M. G. E. & Lopez, R. E. O. (2010). Down syndrome and automatic processing of familiar and unfamiliar emotional faces. *International Journal of Special Education, 25(3),* 17-23.

Lopez, R. E. O. (2009). *Emociones: sobre la naturaleza y función cognitiva de la emoción humana*. México: Trillas

Lubec, G. (2003). *The brain in Down syndrome (trisomy 21)*. Retrieved April 13, 2004, from http://www.altonweb.com/cs/downsyndrome/lubec.html.

Lund, N. (2001). *Attention and pattern recognition*. New York, NY, EE. UU.: Taylor and Francis Inc.

Matsumoto, D., LeRoux, J., Wilson- Cohn, C., Raroque J., Kooken, K., Ekman, P. & Goh, A. (2000). A new test to measure emotion recognition ability: Mastsumoto and Ekman's japanese and caucasian brief affect recognition test (JACBART). *Journal of Nonverbal Behaviour, 24*(3), 179-209. doi: 10.1023/A:1006668120583

Mondloch, C. J., Lewis, T., Budreau, R., Maurer, D., Dannemiller, J., Stephens, B. & Kleiner-Gathercoal, K. (1999). Face preference during early infancy. *Psychology Science, 10*(5), 419-422. doi: 10.1111/1467-9280.00179

Morales, M. G. E. & Lopez, R. E. O. (2012). Down syndrome and emotional face recognition from a connectionist point of view. *Revista Mexicana de Psicología Educativa (RMPE), 1*(2), 41-53

Morales, M. G. E. & Lopez, R. E. O. (2005). Mecanismos cognitivos de reconocimiento de información emocional en personas con síndrome de Down. *Revista Médica Internacional sobre Síndrome de Down, 9*(1), 2-6.

Morales, M. G. E. & Lopez, R. E. O. (2006). El síndrome de Down y su mundo emocional [The emotional world of Down's syndrome]. Mexico: Trillas.

Morales, M. G. E. & Lopez, R. E. O. (2011). El reconocimiento facial emocional en el síndrome de Down: modelando desde una perspectiva conexionista. *Revista Mexicana de Psicología Educativa 1*(2), 41-53.

Morales, M. G. E., & Lopez, R. E. O. (2010). Down syndrome and automatic processing of familiar and unfamiliar emotional faces. *International Journal of Special Education, 25(3),* 17-23. Retrieved from http://www.eric.ed.gov/ERICWebPortal/search/recordDetails.jsp?ERICExtSearch_SearchValue_0=EJ909032&searchtype=keyword&ERICExtSearch_SearchType_0=no&_pageLabel=RecordDetails&accno=EJ909032&_nfls=false&source=ae

Morales, M. G. E. (2004). *Mecanismos cognitivos de reconocimiento de información emocional en personas con síndrome de Down*. (Master theses unpublished, Universidad Autónoma de Nuevo Leon, Monterrey, México).

Morales, M. G. E., Charles, C. D. J. & Lopez, R. E. O. (2008). Actitudes hacia los maestros, emociones académicas y mecanismos cognitivos de evaluación emocional de los estudiantes [Ungraduate student's the attitude toward teacher, academic emotions and cognitive mechanisms of emotional appraisal]. En N. L. Pérez (Ed.). *La voz de los investigadores en Psicología Educativa: dos cuerpos académicos en red.* México: Ediciones cultura de Veracruz.

Morales, M. G. E., Lopez, R. E. O. & Hedlefs, A. M. I. (2010). *La expresión facial como una revelación de la emoción y el pensamiento.* México: Trillas

Morton, J., &. Johnson, M. H. (1991). Conspec and conlern a two-process theory of infant face recognition. *Psychologycal Review, 98*(2), 164-181. doi: 10.1037/0033-295X.98.2.164

Musch, J. & Klauer, K. C. (Eds.) (2003). *The psychology of evaluation: Affective processes in cognition and emotion* (pp. 109-137). Mahthaw, NJ., EE. UU.: LEA

Oveis, C., Gruber, J., Keltner, D., Stamper, J. L. & Boyce, W. T. (2009). Smile intensity and warm touch as thin slices of child and family affective style. *Emotion, 9*(4), 544–548. doi: 10.1037/a0016300

Papageorgiou, C. & Wells, A. (2004). *Depressive Rumination: Nature, theory and treatment.* England: John Wiley & Sons Ltd.

Parkin, A. (1999). *Exploraciones en neuropsicología cognitiva*. Madrid: Médica Panamericana.

Parrish, J. (2007). *Affective priming and memory for faces and semantic information.* (Dissertation Abstracts International, 68(03), Microfilms de la Rosalind Franklin University of Medicine and Science, Chicago, Illinois, EE.UU). Retrieved from http://proquest.umi.com/pqdlink?Ver=1&Exp=12-29-2017&FMT=7&DID=1306876011&RQT=309&attempt=1&cfc=1 (AAT 3258312)

Pine, D. S., Lissek, S., Klein, R. G., Mannuzza, S. Moulton, J. L., Guardino, M. & Woldehawariat, G. (2004). Face-memory and emotion: associations with major depression in children and adolescents. *Journal of Child Psychology and Psychiatry, 45*(7), 1199–1208. doi: 10.1111/j.1469-7610.2004.00311.x

Pitcairn, T. & Wishart, J. (2000). Face processing in Children With Down Syndrome. En D. Weeks, R. Chua & D. Elliot (Eds.). *Perceptual-Motor behaviour in Down syndrome* (pp. 123-147). Edinburgh, Inglaterra: Human Kinetics.

Plutchik, R. (1994). *The psychology and biology of emotion*. New York, NY, EE. UU.: Harper Collins College Publishers.

Pollak, S. & Kistler, D. (2002). Early experience is associated with the development of categorical representations for facial expressions of emotion. *PNAS, 99*(13), 9072-9076. Retrieved from http://www.pnas.org/content/99/13/9072.full.pdf

Porter, M., Coltheart, M. & Langdon, R. (2007). The neuropsychological basis of hypersociability in Williams and Down syndrome. *Neuropsychologia*, *45*(12), 2839-2849. Retrieved from http://dx.doi.org/10.1016/j.neuropsychologia.2007.05.006

Prkachin, G. C. (2003). The effect of orientation on detection and identification of facial expression of emotion. British Journal of Psychology, 94, 45-62. doi: 10.1348/000712603762842093

Quinones, I., Pérez, J., Leon, I. & Bobes, A. (2006). Vínculos afectivos y procesamiento de caras: Un estudio con potenciales evocados y fMRI. In E. Gámez & J. M. Díaz (Eds.). *Investigaciones en Psicología Básica ULL: Psicolingüística, Razonamiento y Emoción* (pp. 185 – 195). España: Universidad de la Laguna.

Raz, N., Torres, I. & Briggs, S. D. (1995). Selective neuroanatomical abnormalities in Down's syndrome and their cognitive correlates: Evidence from MRI morphometry. *Neurology, 45*, 356-366.

Reynolds, J. K. & Pezdek, K. (1992). Face recognition memory: The effects of exposure duration and encoding instruction. *Applied Cognitive Psychology, 6*(4), 279-292. Retrieved from http://www.cgu.edu/include/Face_Recognition_Memory.pdf

Rogers, T.T. & McClelland, J. J. (2004). *Semantic cognition: A parallel distributed approach*. Cambridge, Massachusetts: MIT Press.

Russell, J. A. & Fher, B. (1987). Relativity in the perception of emotion in facial expressions. *Journal of Experimental Psychology: General, 116*(3), 223-237. doi: 10.1037/0096-3445.116.3.223

Scherer, K. R. (2001). Appraisal considered as a process of multilevel sequential checking. En K. R. Scherer, A. Schorr & T. Johnstone (Eds.). *Appraisal processes in emotion: theory, methods, research* (pp, 92-120). Nueva York, NY, EE. UU.: Oxford University Press.

Scherer, K. R. (1987). Toward a dynamic theory of emotion: The component process model of affective states. *Geneva Studies in Emotion and Communication*, *1*, 1-98. Retrieved August 19, 2004, from http://www.unige.ch/fapse/emotion/genstudies/genstudies.html

Schorr, A. (2001). Subjective measurement in appraisal research: Present state and future perspectives. En K. R. Scherer, A. Schorr & T. Johnstone (Eds.). *Appraisal processes in emotion: theory, methods, research* (pp, 331-349). New York, NY, EE. UU.: Oxford University Press.

Schwarzer, G. (2000). Development of face processing: the effect of face inversion. *Child Development, 71*(2), 391-401. Retrieved from http://infantlab.fiu.edu/Articles/Schwarzer%202000.pdf

Schwarzer, G., Zauner, N. & Korell, M. (2003). Face processing during the first decade of life. En G. Schwarzer & H. Leder (Eds.). *The development of face processing* (pp. 55-68). EE. UU.: Hogrefe & Huber Publishers.

Bouras N., Turk, J. & Cornish, K. (1998). Face recognition and emotion perception in boys with Fragile X syndrome. *Journal of Intellectual Disability Research, 42*(6), 490-499. doi: 10.1046/j.1365-2788.1998.4260490.x

Valentine, T. (1988). Upside-down faces: A review of the effect of inversion upon face recognition. *British Journal of Psychology, 79*, 471-491. doi: 10.1111/j.2044-8295.1988.tb02747.x

Valentine, T. (1995). *Cognitive and computational aspects of face recognition: Explorations in face space*. New York: Routledge.

Van der Geest, J. N., Kemner, C., Verbaten, M. N. & van England, H. (2002). Gaze behaviour of children with pervasive developmental disorder toward human faces: a fixation time study. *Journal of Child Psychology and Psychiatry, 43*(5), 669-678.

Wang, P. P., Doherty, S. Rourkc, S. B. & Bellugi, U. (1995). Unique profile of visuoperceptual skills in genetic syndrome. *Brain and Cognition, 29*(1), 54-65. Retrieved from http://lcn.salk.edu/publications/1995/Wang%20-%20Unique%20profile%201995.pdf

Williams, K. R., Wishart, J. G., Pitcairn, T. K. & Willis, D. S. (2005). Emotion recognition by children with Down syndrome: investigation of specific impairments and error profiles. *American Journal on Mental Retardation, 110*(5), 378-392. Retrieved from http://www.aaiddjournals.org/doi/abs/10.1352/0895-8017%282005%29110%5B378%3AERBCWD%5D2.0.CO%3B2

Wishart, J. & Pitcairn, T. (2000). Recognition of identity and expression in faces by children with Down syndrome. *American Journal on Mental Retardation, 105*(6), 466-479. Retrieved from http://www.aaiddjournals.org/doi/abs/10.1352/0895-8017%282000%29105%3C0466%3AROIAEI%3E2.0.CO%3B2

Wishart, J. G., Cebula, K. R., Willis, D. S. & Pitcairn, T. K. (2007). Understanding of facial expressions of emotion by children with intellectual disabilities of differing aetiology. *Journal of Intellectual Disability Research, 51*(7), 551-563. doi: 10.1111/j.1365-2788.2006.00947.x

Zebrowitz, L. A. (2006). Finally, faces find favor. *Social Cognition, 24*(5), 657-701. doi: 10.1521/soco.2006.24.5.657

Chapter 4

Envisioning an Amazing Emotional World: The Down Syndrome Case of Happiness, Love, Pain and Blame

Abstract

Human emotional life is complex and sometimes paradoxical, since deep in our brains two emotional realities seem to coexist. First, a positive emotional system provides people the capacity to feel things like closeness, and thus to feel the need to approach other people, or to experience attachment or satisfaction, among other possible desirable experiences. On the other side, a negative emotional system provides psychological and behavioural mechanisms for avoidance, protection or fighting for survival. With an understanding of the dynamic and emergent interaction between both emotional systems during atypical development (e.g. DS), it is possible to devise improvements to the quality of life inside the population with DS. Following this direction, we will next briefly discuss how members of this population perceive and experience positive emotions (e.g. happiness and love) as well as their counterpart: negative emotions (e.g. pain). Moreover, we will also review how the DS emotional system constrains higher cognitive processing when members of this population are required to perform moral reasoning.

4.1. Down Syndrome and Positive Emotion Human System

Happiness and its pursuit typify an essential part of the human experience. If you have ever met a person with DS you probably remember her/him among the happiest persons you have ever known. After noticing this, one might wonder if they experience happiness the same way as the rest of us do. Certainly, careful observation of how members of this population express this particular emotion allows us to identify some differences in their emotional behaviour. Unfortunately, not many academic explorations in current emotion theory or special education research on DS and happiness can be obtained, and as we will discuss next, only a few academic asides provide insights about how and why many persons with this genetic condition characterize themselves as happy people. In addressing this here, we will consider one of the most important conversation topics for young and adult people with DS, namely, love and romantic relationships. This approach is meant to empower a discussion on love in terms of an emotion circumscribed to happiness inside this population, and at the same time is meant to suggest a new research direction to explore: whether we misjudge their ability to be responsible for to have family and offspring. Thus, one final goal of this chapter is to provide research-based suggestions to improve their lives by considering differences between how they and we perceive happiness and love.

4.2. Down Syndrome: A Happy Existence or Just an Illusion?

> "I see persons with DS always as children. They are innocent, without any kind of evil, they never hurt anyone else...,"
>
> Anonymous mom of person with DS

There is a belief among parents and special education teachers that suggests a DS common identity that entails less diversity than that found in a typical population (Wishart & Johnston, 1990). Specifically, members of this population have been typified as stubborn and not easygoing (Dykens, Shah, Sagun, Beck & King, 2002). On the other hand they have been typified as having a great sense of humor (Down, 1866), highly emotional (Smith & Walden, 1998), very tender and affectionate (Lecavalier & Tasse, 2005), fun to be with (Hodapp, 2001), and relentlessly "happy children" (Robison, 2000).

It is our strongest belief that this last observation regarding happiness constitutes a DS continuous and distinctive trait. However, due to their genetic condition several questions arise regarding whether or not the way they experience happiness (or other positive emotions) is the same way as we do. Is it true they are happier than typical individuals? How do they experience positive emotions? What are the emotional differences between typical persons and people with DS regarding positive emotions? Let us discuss by first considering emotion theory and happiness, and then a circumscribed emotion of happiness: Love.

4.2.1. Some Remarks on Happiness

It does not matter if the pursuit of happiness is genetically driven or learned, or both (e.g., Lykken, 2000; Layard, 2005; Lykken & Tellegen, 1996; Veenhoven, 1991), the achievement of such an emotional goal has an impact on the way we adapt to our environment and social context (e.g., marriage, friendship, income, work performance, etc.; Lyubomirsky, King & Diener, 2005) as well as on our health (there is a documented relation between positive emotions and our immunological system; Pettit, Kline, Gencoz, Gencoz, & Joiner, 2001).

However, even though hundreds of books have been written on happiness and there are few of us who have not experienced this emotion, the truth is, its meaning and emotional nature remains far from clear (Lu, 2001). Conceptualizations of happiness range from the spiritual domain, to behavioural definitions or just as an emotion with its own psychological dimensions (see Table 4.1).

Table 4.1. Some sample definitions of happiness

	Definitions
Veenhoven (1984)	*"Happiness is the degree to which an individual's overall evaluation of his life as a whole, concludes positively. As such, happiness is an experience that only creatures of consciousness can undergo. It is an essentially experiential phenomenon which cannot be identified with particular external conditions or with a way of life".*
(Veenhoven, 1991, p. 2)	*"Happiness is conceived here as the degree to which an individual judges the overall quality of his life favorably". "Happiness can also be called 'life-satisfaction'. When this evaluation of life crystallizes into a stable view, we can speak of happiness as an 'attitude' towards one's life".*
(Lu, 2001, p. 407)	*"Happiness can be defined in terms of a mental state of satisfaction and contentment; positive feelings/emotions; a harmonious homeostasis; achievement and hope; and freedom from ill-being". "Happiness is a harmonious state of existence, under the following conditions: the individual is satisfied or content; the individual is the agent of his own happiness; spiritual enrichment is emphasized more than material satisfaction; and the individual maintains a positive outlook for the future".*
Layard (2003, p.4)	*"By happiness I mean feeling good – enjoying life and feeling it is wonderful".*
(Argyle, 2001, p. 22)	"Happiness is found to be a single factor of experience, but it consists of at least three partly independent factors- satisfaction with life, positive affect and negative affect".

Due to the wide variety of academic definitions of happiness, some recommendations suggest that its definition must include at least operative terms like 1) Positive affect, 2) life satisfaction index, 3) absence of negative affect (Lu, 2001) and 4) a theoretical distinction of happiness from other positive emotions.

Considering these set guidelines, it has been suggested that positive emotions of joy, exhilaration, ecstasy, and so on are mostly transitory or short-term emotions whereas happiness can be circumscribed to a long-term mood state (Power & Dalgleish, 2008). Even thus, positivity and happiness are interwoven emotional systems, and their interaction affects our psychological well-being. Individuals typified by intense episodes of positivity are characterized as enthusiastic, energetic, confident, and alert. In contrast, those persons having low positive affectivity report substantially reduced levels of happiness, excitement, vigor, and confidence (Watson, 2004).

Furthermore, emotions like joy, exhilaration, ecstasy, etc., are frequently related to the achievement of a particular goal (they have an object) and occupy a high state of consciousness. These do not equal happiness (e.g. it is possible to experience joy with specific goal while not being generally happy). On the other hand, moods like happiness are typically free-floating or objectless, at the background of consciousness (Fredrickson, 2002; Oatley & Jenkins, 1996). Another important distinction is made between it and drives such as satiation of food, thirst, sex, etc., which relate more to a dimension of pleasure rather than happiness.

In terms of cognitive behaviour, positive emotions are assumed to broaden the range of available thought–actions, such as encouraging play, exploration, and creative thinking (Isen, 1999). Thus, positive moods relate to non-specific/global judgments (Fredrickson, 2005), and happiness seems to be the more global holistic positive experience. In contrast, negative emotions such as sadness, anger, or disgust are circumscribed to local or focalized judgments associated with specific behaviours. Take as an example, fear once it is generated by a personal appraisal, a limited range of behaviours like running, fighting or freezing are then available.

The positive and negative affective systems are considered different emotional dimensions, but which still belong to a global goal-oriented behaviour system. Thus, whereas the negative affect underlies the withdrawal-oriented behavioural inhibition system, the positive affect is a component of the approach-oriented behavioural facilitation system, guiding people toward pleasure and reward situations and experiences leading to happiness. Reported experiences in ratios of positive to negative emotions in healthy individuals suggest a typical proportion of 3:1 (Fredrickson, 2005). However, higher positive over negative ratios have been obtained from functional individuals (Schwartz, 1992). In general, Power and Dalgleish (2008) suggest that healthy positive individuals are characterized by at least:

a) Having a basic memory bias for positive material
b) The tendency of the cognitive system to maintain positive affect.
c) The association between the use of stereotypes in processing and the existence of positive affect.

Some backing for these assertions can be obtained from affective priming research. Studies from this academic field have suggested that typical individuals with no emotional disorders tend to automatically process positive emotion faster than neutral and negative information, whereas depressed or anxious people tend to process negative or stressful information faster (Figure 4.1). Apparently, people who explicitly report to be moderately happy have a brain tuned to immediately process positive information, whereas processing negative information requires more cognitive participation (perhaps as a better way to cope with bad behavioural consequences).

As was discussed in Chapter 3, people with DS also present an automatic cognitive emotional bias toward faster recognition of positive information. However, their appraisal processing of positive information seems to be particularly remarkable, and qualitatively different from the typical population. Let us further explore on this last observation by presenting some examples and academic findings regarding people with DS's positive affection and conceptualization of happiness.

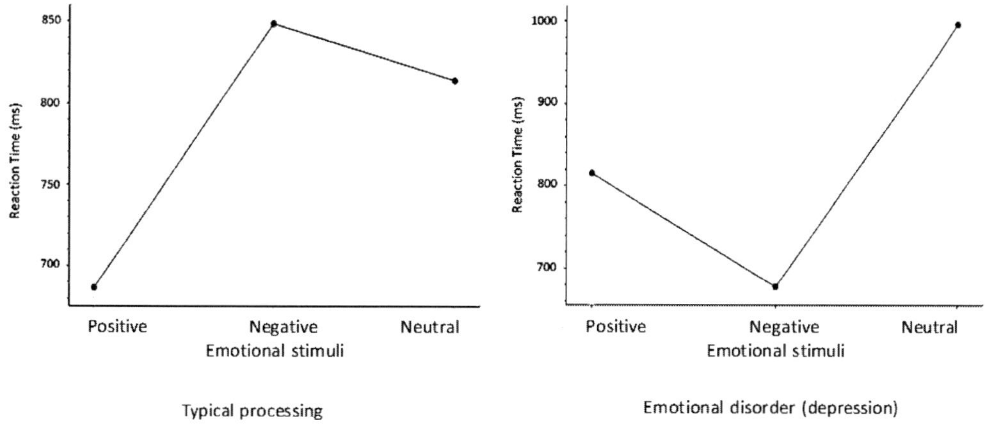

Figure 4.1. Typical automatic appraisal of emotional information (top) is biased to recognize positive information faster than negative or neutral information. The opposite is true for people with a depressive emotional disorder (bottom).

4.2.2. People with DS and Happiness

Interviewer: When is it that you feel happy?
Young adult with DS: I have been happy for many years....
Interviewer: Can you give me an example of a time when you feel happy?
Young adult with DS: I am happy now.
Interviewer: Exactly, why?
Young adult with DS: How can I explain it to you?
Interviewer: Explain it to me any way you want, when is it that you are happy?
Young adult with DS: All my life.

This interview fragment is interesting because it provides specific information about how this young adult perceives himself (happy all his life). Yes, but is it possibly for a human to always be happy? Well, a tiny Himalayan kingdom called Bhutan not only promotes that this concept should be possible but that it must be a global agenda. Contrary to the idea that increasing national economy wealth leads people to increased happiness, Bhutan's government has been designed to promote happiness as the main engine for increasing social progress and national welfare. In fact, Bhutan was the first country to propose a happiness index in 1972 (The Gross National Happiness; GNH).

Unfortunately, according to the World Happiness Report (Helliwell, Layard & Sachs, 2012) the highest happiness and life satisfaction value indexes were reported by Denmark, Finland, and other northern European countries, not Bhutan. Instead, the GNH Index value obtained by Bhutan in 2010 was 0.737, which means that only 40.8% of the people had achieved happiness (profoundly happy and extensively happy), while the remaining 59% were reported to be slightly happy or unhappy.

One immediately wonders about why a GNH-oriented government is not able to achieve the highest satisfaction and happiness index values. Some criticism to the GNH program emphasizes that happiness indexes are subjective and biased by private political considerations and thus other countries score better than others. Some argue that until there is a complete definition of what happiness accounts for, there is no sense in measuring which is the happiest country (McCloskey, 2012).

As suggested by Helliwell et al. (2012), happiness has many connotations and its conceptualization is a personal affair. Even those who go through many adverse situations in their lives are capable of feeling happiness. Thus, relevant factors to happiness are many, including genetic considerations, coping strategies to social adaptation, and other personal resources (Lyubomirsky et al., 2005; Lyubomirsky 2007). For instance, a set of genetic research studies on twins suggest that happiness profiles in this population varies according to genetic considerations (DeNeve, Christakis, Fowler & Frey, in press). Exactly why this is possible still remain unclear, however it is recognized that hereditary constraints affect susceptibility to emotional disorders (Craddock & Forty, 2006,), resilience capacity (Stein, Campbell-Sills & Gelernter, 2009), personality (Penke, Denissen & Miller, 2007), etc.

In this sense atypical DS genetic conditions represent a window with which to observe how genetic factors may affect our positive emotional system. First, members with DS have a clearly identified etiology (additional genetic material like the chromosome 21), which is associated with specific personality and behavioural factors, as well as with physical and medical characteristics that differentiate them from other intellectual disability groups (Hodapp, 2001). The idea of a specific DS phenotype is not new and since 1866 Langdon Down characterized people with DS with a specific personality type: "*They have considerable power of imitation, even bordering on being mimics. They are humorous, and a lively sense of the ridiculous often colours their mimicry...*". Even when there is still a debate over the existence of a DS phenotype, it is clear that regarding emotional behaviour they tend to send more positive messages than normal (Fidler, 2005), smile more frequently (Fidler, Barrett & Most, 2005), have more positive affection (Capps, Kasari, Yirmiya, & Sigman, 1993) and show more pro-social behaviour (Kasari, Freeman, & Bass, 2003).

It is not clear if this positive personality image is directly or indirectly related to their genetic condition, but is clear that genetic factors are related to their "baby face" or angelical facial display even as adults. This physical appearance promotes more affectionate and loving interactions from parents and family (Hodapp, 2001). Take for instance a study where mothers with children with DS reported less stressful relations than mothers having children with another kind of disability. They reported their relations as acceptable and reinforcing (Hodapp, Ricci, Ly, & Fidler, 2003). This is a general perception, and does not necessarily apply to every DS case. However, this generally positive view is reinforced by the aforementioned DS self-perception of being happy people. Consider as another example the study carried by Skotko, Levine and Goldstein (2011), where 99% of 284 persons with DS self-described as very happy individuals. Similar results were obtained when participants from previously described affective priming studies (Chapter 3) were required to list the most common emotions in their life. As expected, participants most identified with positive emotions (happy or very happy). Here, 9 out of 15 participants with DS stated that at the time they felt very happy, 4 reported feeling some happiness, 1 being pleasant or comfortable and just one sad. After the same participants were required to describe the second most common emotion they experienced, the emotion range was reduced to fear and anger, (positive emotions reports were minor). Not all participants reported a second or third most experienced emotion (see Figure 4.2.)

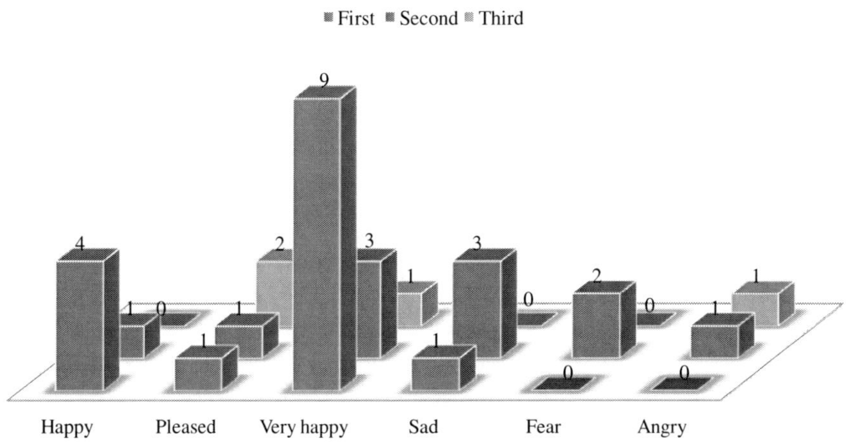

Figure 4.2. The number of participants with DS that reported feeling a specific emotion. First row columns (from the front to back) describe the participants' most common emotion. The second row indicates the second most relevant emotion and so on.

It is important not to misread these results. Most typical individuals (in smaller frequency and intensity) also have a tendency to be positive or happy, whether living with some physical limitation (like quadriplegia) or low income (Diener & Diener, 1996). However, the question remains as to whether people with DS share the same psychological nature to be happy as typical individuals.

It has been suggested that economic factors, contextual variables (such as politics, religion, labor conditions, etc.), relational conditions (with a romantic partner, friends or family) as well as personal characteristics (like self esteem, sense of control, optimism, personal freedom among others) affect a person's level of happiness (Changrian, 2010). As it similar concerns can be observed in people with DS (again, referring to participants from previous affective priming studies).

Note in Table 4.2 that happiness was the emotion that produced the bigger events set. These events related more to activities than to objects. This is congruent with some results reported by a study from Wuang & Su (2012) where teenagers with DS related happiness to informal enjoyment habits such as reading, video games, etc. as well as social enrollment.

A detailed review of Table 4.2 allows us to identify related topics as the most important reasons to be happy. Notice that descriptions of familiar relationships produced more emotional definitions than romantic or friendship relationships. It is hard to infer from this simple interview process whether or not these relationship differences constitute a reality to this population, and more qualified research is needed. However, from the evidence of this simple interview, the important role that interpersonal relationships play (friendship, love, etc.) can be inferred. This relational activity is assumed relevant for emotional development and general well being. As was suggested by Veenhoven (1991, p. 1): "*People cannot be happy in chronic hunger, danger and isolation: not even if they have never known better and if their neighbours are worse off...*".

Table 4.2. Some reasons why study participants with DS may feel happiness, sadness or fear

Happiness	Sadness	Anger	Fear
Playing on the street	I was hit	Physician	When I see Chucky
Now, friends and family	To see my mother crying	My ugly and foolish brother makes me angry	Fear when I see a rat
When I received my iPad as a gift	Sad, because I misbehave		
Details in a letter	My grandfather died		
Reading books	My dad died		
Being congratulated			
Happy when I see my friends			
Happy when I receive a present			
Happy because there are women			
I have a lover			
Glad to see my girlfriend			
When I am with my parents, grandparents, cousins, my uncle.			
Old, on my birthday I was happy.			
When I talk to my sisters			
When I am home			
Restroom			
When I watch TV because I see my boyfriend			
I love to paint, I enjoy painting			
I am happy if you are happy too			
I felt I am happy at Christmastime			
Surfing the internet, eating cookies			

* The list of 15 participants with DS' responses to the question of what makes them happy, feel angry, sad or being afraid. The partcipants belong to different Mexican communities.

Accordingly, by exploring the way people with DS perceive relational information, we can not only modify current stereotypes about their prosocial behaviour but also understand more specificities regarding the way they conceive happiness. This is particularly important in the case of their romantic relationships. On the one hand, heated debates about their rights to enroll in formal romantic relationships, to have offspring or a family by their own, have limited their quality of life. Lack of knowledge about their romantic needs have even equated their concept of love to the level of sexual intercourse. As we will discuss next, these conceptions are based on misconceptions about DS romantic relations and happiness. On the other hand, determining the emotional and cognitive nature of DS romantic behaviour will lead to the establishment of academic guidelines by which they may improve their quality of life (a basic necessity of being loved), as well as to encourage new research to better understand the cognitive nature underlying DS social approaching behaviour and happiness.

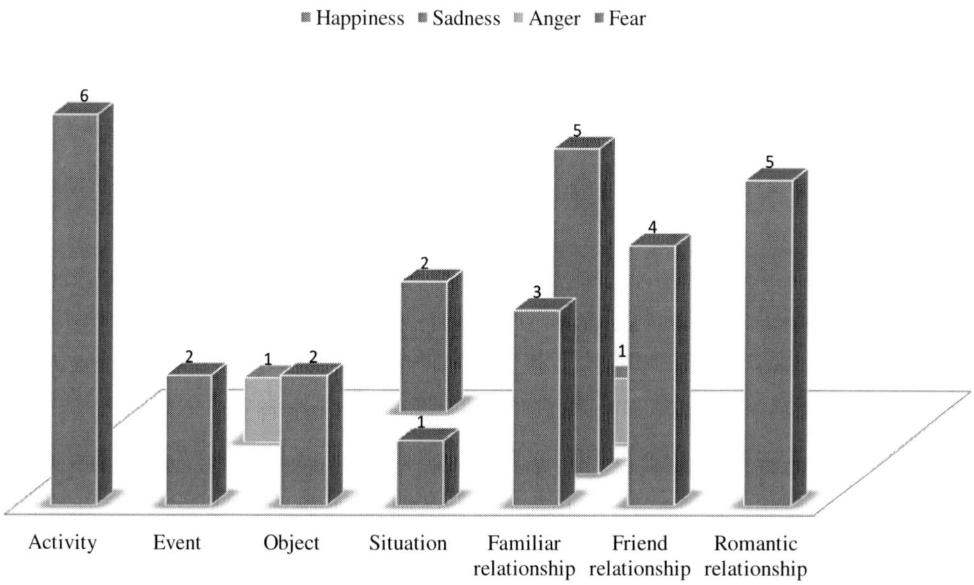

Figure 4.3. Number of participants with DS that reported feeling a specific emotion (blue for happiness, red for sadness, green for anger and purple for fear) due to a particular reason (performing an activity, having an interpersonal relationship with family, friends or romantic partner, as well as experiencing a situation, or receiving something valuable to them).

4.3. The Down Syndrome Heart: Love

> "Love is an important matter.... my boyfriend buys me chocolates, cookies, serenades me, takes me to restaurants...."
>
> Young girl with DS

The capacity to experience and give love is fundamental to human development. From very early in our lives, and throughout our entire life, love manifestations mold our identity, our sense of belongingness, the meaning we possess of our life (Murstein, 1988), and influences our interpersonal relationships, our well being and happiness (Arias, Ovejero, & Morentin, 2009, Myers, Sweeney, & Witmer, 2000).

Without any doubt love is one of the biggest human experiences, and people with DS are no exception. If you have ever been in contact with members of this population you will find that a favorite conversation topic of any youngster or an adult with DS relates to love and getting married. Trying to understand love under atypical development is relevant to putting away negative myths, and addressing their rights to get married, sexual intercourse and offspring.

Our current analysis on love science is by no means comprehensive. Only simple theoretical considerations are introduced to frame the capacity of people with DS to get involved in an informal or formal romantic relationship. Rather, consideration of love as a positive emotional style observed in most persons with DS (see chapter 3) will guide the following discussion about their capacity for loving someone else.

4.3.1. A Selected Background on Love

Shining over all other human emotions is the emotional state called love. Even when we can recognize that someone else or even oneself is under the influence of this powerful emotion, a problem arises whenever we try to define it. For some (e.g. Chinese culture) it be seen as as a kind of sadness or other negative emotions such as in the case of "unrequited love", "nostalgia" or "sorrow love" (Shaver, Wu & Schwartz, 1991). It has also been defined as a bitter-sweet experience (1979) and even as a mental illness (Tallis, 2004) due to associated physical and mental discomfort. Furthermore, some negative emotions are strongly related to love, such as shyness, jealousy, anger and insecurity.

On the other hand, love seems to be something worth fighting for. Innumerable positive statements about it exist regarding companionship, happiness, family, sex, and sublime moral emotions that emphasize the positive nature of love. An immense and sometimes exquisite literary work has been written under this view as a living testimony of our insatiable addiction to it. Due to its complexity and sometimes its contradictory nature, love cannot be considered as a single unified concept. As such, love appears to be constrained by a combination of elements or components. Take for instance Lee's love colors model, where three primary styles of love can be combined to create emerging secondary love styles.

Figure 4.4. shows the combinatorial property of this model, in which each possible cell combination of love component translates into a specific love manifestation (Lee 1972; Laswell & Laswell 1976; Hendrick & Hendrick, 1986; Neto, 1993, 1994).

In this model, Pragma love relates to social conventions (e.g considering parents approval over a romantic partner) whereas Agape and Mania love are identified as internal emotions regulating the relationship between a couple. Neto and colleagues (2000) have presented empirical support of this model in a number of cultures.

Rather than trying to completely describe Lee's love colors model, let us emphasize the componential property assigned to it. This property is widely disseminated through different approaches studying the study of love, including one of the most influential theories of love, the so-called triangular theory. In this theory, Sternberg (1986, 1988) visualizes love as composed of three dimensions: intimacy, passion and commitment. Different expressions or types of love emerge from the combination of these dimensions as shown in Figure 4.5.

The passion dimension is associated with a person's sexual drive, whereas commitment and intimacy are related to forms of attachment. Note that some equivalence might be found between Sternberg and Lee's models. For instance, compassionate love from the triangular model resembles Lee's concept of storge (e.g. love from parents to a child) whereas the passion component from Sternberg's model equals the Eros component in Lee's model.

In neither daily life, nor in the time that a romantic relationship endures, is the existence of a static or definite love triangle structure assumed. Rather, the triangular love theory implies that in a relationship, a couple may experience the absence of love (none of the three components), infatuated love (passion only), companionate love (intimacy and commitment), romantic love (intimacy and passion) or the presence of all three components (consummate love).

	EROS ROMANTIC LOVE, PASSIONATE	LUDUS PLAYING GAMES	STORGE FRIENDSHIP
EROS ROMANTIC LOVE, PASSIONATE		MANIA POSSESSIVE LOVE, DEPENDENCY	AGAPE SELFLESS LOVE
LUDUS PLAYING GAMES	MANIA POSSESSIVE LOVE, DEPENDENCY		PRAGMA LOGICAL LOVE
STORGE FRIENDSHIP	AGAPE SELFLESS LOVE	PRAGMA LOGICAL LOVE	

Figure 4.4. Lee's love model describes six love styles. Possible combinations from three primary love styles produce second-order love styles.

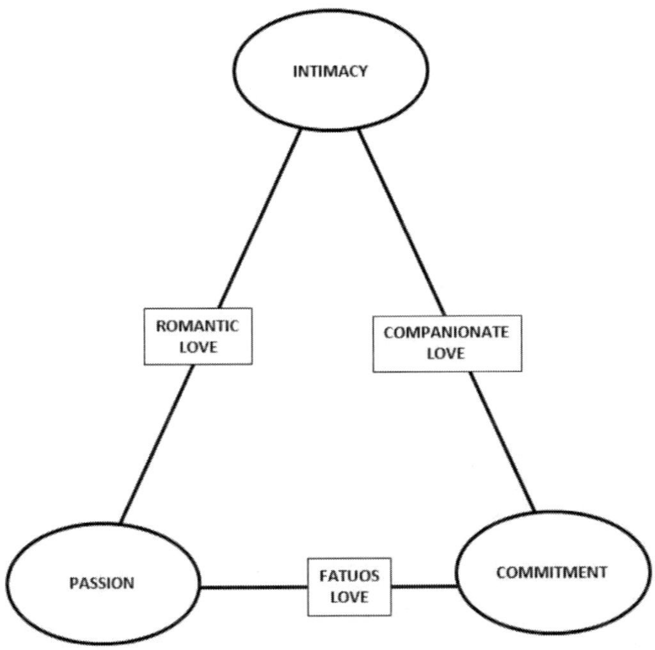

Figure 4.5. Triangular theory of love (Sternberg, 1986, 1988).

Furthermore, romantic partners' valuation of each love component inside a relationship may change, depending on situational romantic factors. This in turn might lead to the development of romantic coping strategies. For example, it might be the case where a couple feels that passion has dangerously decreased, and because of this they decide to increase their relationship commitment (perhaps deciding to have offspring). Interestingly, the way typical development (TD) people evaluate changes in love components in a romantic relationship follows a systematic rule. In particular, Falconi and Mullet (2003) suggest that systematic dynamic changes of love components are best described using the following equation:

Love = f (w_P Passion * w_I Intimacy * w_C Commitment)

where W_s expresses the weight of each component in a given love relationship.

By using an Information Integration Theory (IIT) approach to the subject (see next section in this chapter) these authors present empirical support for an exponential function relating to perceived love and the degree of passion. This approach to studying how romantic partners perceive love allows quantitative specification for degrees of change in each component through different situational romantic scenarios. For example, in their study of love through the adult life, they found some support to the common belief that elderly participants perceive increased commitment as well as a decrease in passion. However, the researchers were capable to determine that passion is the most important factor in any age, followed by intimacy and commitment.

Academic evidence for a componential and dimensional human love structure has been a theoretical watershed on the study of human romantic relationships. Additional information about how love components interact and integrate (through algebraic rules) to cope with romantic relationships allows for some behavioural predictions inside romantic relationships. However, as we are about to discuss, not much is known about DS romantic activity, and only theoretical interpolations can be made using the scarce academic love research dealing with DS.

4.3.2. Love and Down Syndrome from Integration Information Theory Point of View

In terms of what concerns a triadic love model, there is some evidence suggesting its existence inside intellectual disability populations. For instance, Morentin, Arias, Verdugo, & Rodriguez-Mayoral (2006) studied 75 persons with IDa by having them take Sternberg's triadic love test, from which they obtained evidence for each love component inside the population. Moreover, Morentin et al. (2006) found that people with ID seem to romantically conceptualize the passion love component. Convergent results from another love study with a sample of 376 ID participants (Arias et al., 2009) showed a triadic love structure in this population: Compromise (stability and idealization), passion (physiological arousal), and intimacy (romanticism).

Even when these results do not highlight a specific population with ID, it is clear that there is a possibility of people with DS having a triadic love structure. For example, Table 4.4. shows some people with DS' interview responses to the question: What is love?

Whether these love components are cognitively integrated the same way in a population with DS as in a typical one, remains unknown. A preliminary study on this subject was carried out by Morales, Lopez, Charles and Mullet (2012, abstract). Here, an IIT study was implemented to determine if algebraic integration rules of love factors (e.g. Falconi & Mullet, 2003) could differentiate a DS sample from a typical one in romantic scenarios. Figure 4.6 describes the cognitive processes explored in this study.

In turn, this cognitive functional IIT diagram can be applied to describe people with DS' judgment about love. Consider the scenario in which a young teenager named Lilian is telling us a love story. She is in love with Mike (another teenager with DS) and she feels he likes her back since he always looks for her in his free time, hugs her a lot and sometimes he kisses her

(S_1). He gave her a ring and promised always to love her (S_2). Moreover, Mike talks to her a lot about many things (S_3). All these behavioural factors can be psychologically valuated by Lilian in terms of passion, intimacy and commitment, and then integrated by using a cognitive rule (Figure 4.7).

Table 4.3. Interview responses to the question what is love

Love components	Love is:
Passion	Romantic things
	Foolish details (letters, going out, Kisses)
	Boyfriends
	February the 14th
	Loving her a lot
Intimacy	Giving my heart (trusting)
	Communication
	Thrust
Commitment	Respect a woman (fidelity)
	Respect to all women (no cheating)
	I must respect my romantic partner
	Having a nice family
	Contentment (making the other person happy)

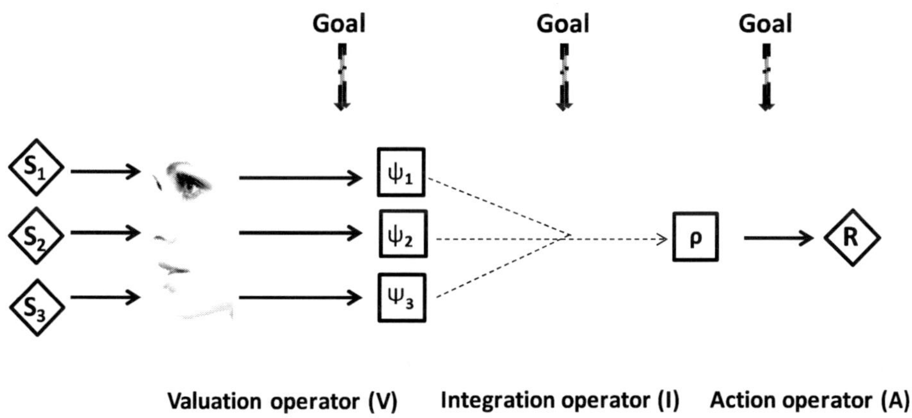

Figure 4.6. The Integration Information Theory diagram shows how relevant stimuli (Si) are extracted from an environment and psychologically represented through a valuation process (V) with cognitive coefficients (ψi). All of these variables will be systematically integrated (I) to form a unified implicit response (ρ) that will produce an explicit response (R) through an action operator (A). Note that all feed forward phase processing is mediated by a goal (see Anderson, 1982).

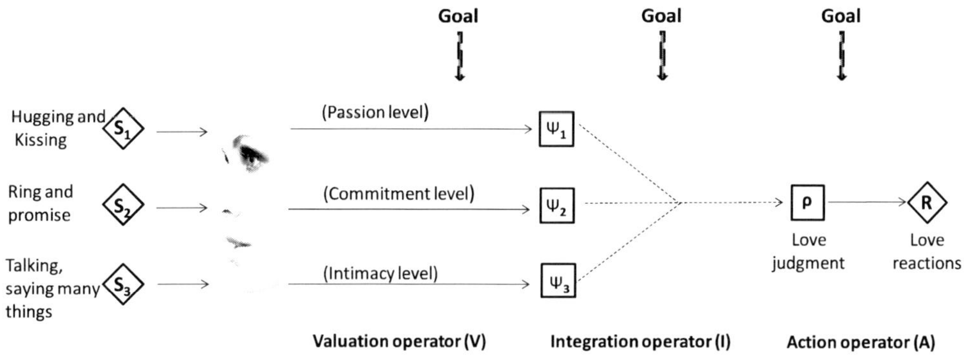

Figure 4.7. This graphic shows the IIT schema extrapolation over a love scenario between two young persons with DS. The three step feed-forward diagram describes how romantic stimuli activate V-I-A cognitive processing, leading to a judgment (ρ) about a romantic partner that is physical expressed (R).

The systematic cognitive behaviour from Figure 4.7. integrating romantic information can be formally described using the following mathematical function:

$$\rho = I(s_1, s_2, s_3)$$

where ρ represents an implicit response that is functionally related to a specific combination (I) of psychological valuated stimuli (s). All elements in the equation cannot be directly observed, but they can be inferred using a careful consideration of direct available information (R, S) that can be measured, numerically quantified and graphically interpreted by cognitive algebra theory.

The cognitive algebra approach assumes that if two or more factors (love and compromise or love and passion) are psychologically integrated using a mathematical rule, then an interaction graph from an experimental design might visually show systematic data organization in a two-dimensional space (Morales, 2012). For example, the use of a summative rule will be reflected as a set of parallel lines such as the ones shown in Figure 4.10. The use of multiplicative rules will be characterized by a linear fan pattern. Average rules can also be distinguished in human cognitive behaviour using crossover patterns (see Anderson, 1982, 1996; also see Neto & Mullet, 1998; Farkas, 1991; Guillet, Hermand & Mullet, 2002; Lazreg and Mullet, 2001).

The IIT approach has provided evidence of the application of these cognitive rules in a variety of behavioural phenomena. For example, ethical behaviour (Frileux, Muñoz-Sastre & Antonini, 2004; Guedj, Gibert, Maudet, Muñoz-Sastre, Mullet & Sorum, 2005; Guedj, Muñoz-Sastre, Mullet & Sorum, 2009), interpersonal relations (Falconi & Mullet, 2003; Farkas, 1991), pleasure obtained from visual and auditory stimuli (Lazreg & Mullet, 2001; Makri & Mullet, 2003) and health matters (Hermand, Mullet & Lavieville, 1997; Muñoz-Sastre, Mullet & Sorum, 1999; Simeone, Hermand & Mullet, 2002).

Love is no exception to this cognitive systematic behaviour (Falconi & Mullet, 2003) and it appears that the same principle applies to persons with atypical development, such as people with DS. Thus, in their study Morales et al. (2012: abstract) found that participants with DS showed *commitment* as the highest valuated love factor followed by the *intimacy* factor, and then passion. These factors were integrated by a summative cognitive rule.

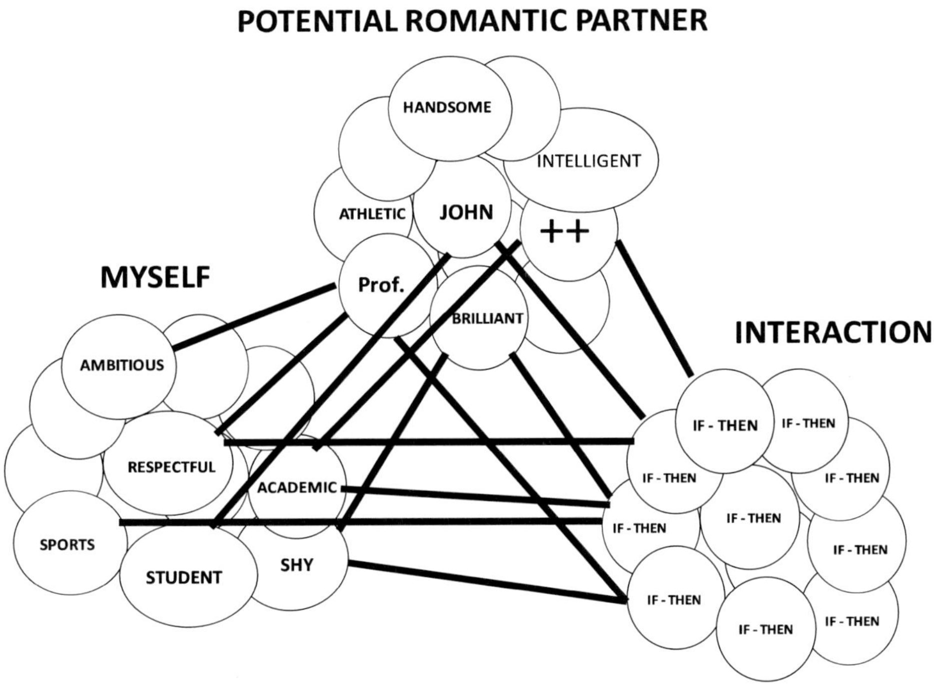

Figure 4.8. A relational schema allows identifying meaningful conditions (if-then) that relate a person to someone else.

Even when these kinds of results represent insightful explorations on how people with DS use romantic functional schemas, more research is needed to understand how this romantic schemata can be applied into DS romantic relationship. As has been pointed out by Beck (1989), formal and informal successful romantic relationships demand from a couple more than just being in love. Well-orchestrated cognitive and emotional functioning is also demanded in order to cope with the dynamic requirements for sustaining a romantic adventure. Proper guidelines or scripts about how to behave and interact with a romantic partner need to be established, and love is just one element (a very important one) inside this relationship script. Baldwin (1992) proposes that these relationship guidelines are learned relationship schemas that are stored in our long-term memory. These romantic schemata refer to cognitive structures about the self, other, and patterns of interpersonal romantic relatedness (Andersen & Cole; Baldwin, Fehr, Keedian, Seidel & Thomson, 1993; Baldwin, Granzberg, Pippus & Pritchard, 2003; Baldwin & Keelan, 1999). Here, simple IF-THEN thinking patterns to elaborate expectancies over a romantic relationship as well as the use of interaction protocols can be elaborated. For example: "If I am successful he will be more interested in me because…" (Figure 4.8).

As we are just about to discuss, this method of emotional valuation of personal attributes (positive or negative), as well as the valuation of non emotional partner's personal attributes might have important implications to persons with DS when they evaluate love components inside their romantic relationships, or when they choose a romantic partner.

4.3.3. Selection of Romantic Partner from DS's Point of View

If you are familiar with the dating behaviour of youth and adults with DS you will observe that they engage in as frequent dating behaviour as TD teenagers and young adult people. How do both populations choose a potential romantic partner? And are the populations significantly different when they have chosen someone to love?

Choosing a romantic partner is a complex event that activates a variety of cognitive processes (Haselton, 2012). It has been suggested that similarity in physical attractiveness, attitudes, believes and moral values are relevant variables in deciding upon a romantic partner (for a theoretical review see Simpson & Gangestad, 2003). Specifically, "unrestricted" people tend to look for people who are physically more attractive, sexually oriented, and have high social distinctiveness, whereas "restricted" people tend look for romantic people, tenderness, and responsible and faithful partners (Simpson & Gangestad, 2003). The above typification statement also seems to apply to people with DS. Table 4.4 shows interview responses from some participants with DS regarding how they choose a potential romantic partner.

As can be seen from Table 4.4, people with DS consider a wide personality attribute spectrum, similar to that of typical persons. These are positive and inclusive attributes.

Regarding the attractiveness statements in the IIT approach, Morales, Charles and Lopez carried on an exploratory study where three different sources of information (Physical appearance, Social personality, Intellectual abilities), were combined in an orthogonal way to generate eight romantic scenarios. Each scenario described a hypothetical and concrete situation with a potential romantic partner. At the end of each scenario, a question was asked about the participant's attractiveness judgment about the person described. Below the question, an adapted 10-point scale response (see frog scale in Morales, 2012) with a "Very attractive" as a right-hand anchor was presented. A possible scenario would go as follows:

Table 4.4. People with DS interview responses to the question: What is you like most when you like a possible girl/boy?

Dimension	Atributte	Peolple with DS's response
Behaviour	Courting	My house (visiting frequently)
		She/he speaks frequently by phone
Emotionality	Easygoing	No yelling, no anger, etc.
	Good mood	Happy
Physical	Similarity	I like they are persons with DS.
		I like people like me (with Down syndrome)
	Attractiveness	Physical: Short (not taller than me)
		Pretty, handsome
		The way they dress
Personality	Faithful	Serious (not a cheater)
	Extroverted and sociable	A talker
		With friends
		Dancer
Global		All the above

"In a meeting you are introduced to a young person with Down syndrome. He is not very handsome and sometimes he is not careful about his physical appearance. He is shy and has a serious personality, he has few friends. Moreover, he is not very clever since he has learning problems and he finds difficult to solve problems. He is not very good at adapting himself to new situations."

As a potential romantic partner, how attractive is this person for you?
o-----o-----o-----o-----o-----o-----o-----o------o-----o Very attractive

Results suggested that for a typical population, intellectual dimensions produced the strongest effect followed by the physical factor and finally the social factor. Participants with ID, however, evaluated the physical appearance factor as the most relevant, followed by the intellectual factor and finally by the social factor (Figure 4.9.). In interviews, the social factor was explicitly reported to be more relevant to persons with ID than typical individuals.

Although the study samples are small, results suggest both samples use a cognitive summative integration information rule, but valuation of factors was different in each. More research is needed to determine if this behaviour is the same in larger population samples (e.g. by increasing N).

The IIT technique can be used in a single-subject design. Analysis of individual differences is relevant to intellectual disability because relevant comparisons (valuation and integration) of a person against his or her own group can then be identified (see Figure 4.10). In this specific case, the participant valuation of person attributes suggests that physical appearance is not as relevant as it was for the group. Notice that this participant presents a summative rule; that is, the most relevant factors seem to contribute independently and linearly in relation to participant's judgment on attractiveness.

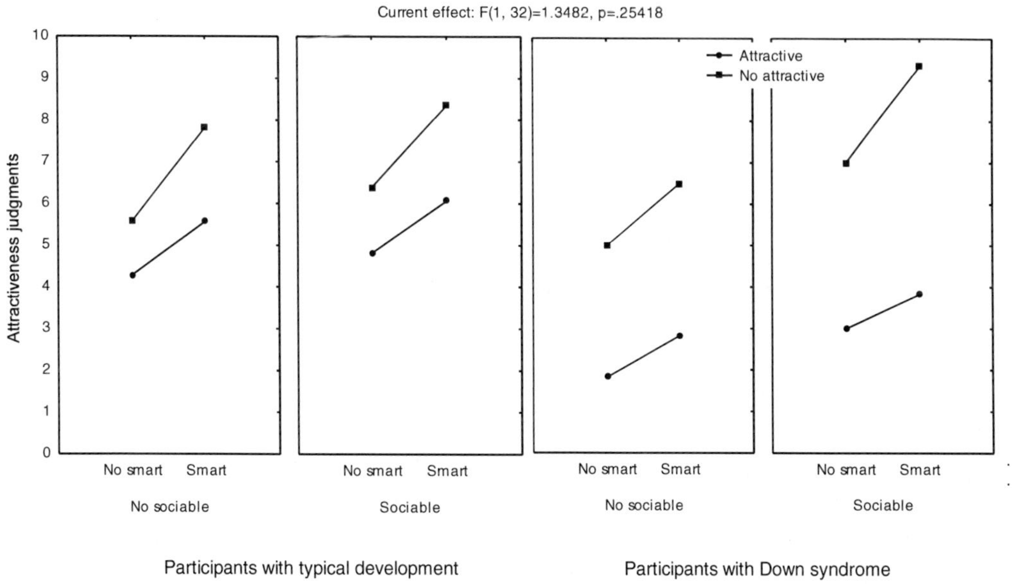

Figure 4.9. These graphs show the interaction effect of Physical appearance, Social personality and Intellectual span on attractiveness judgments for participants with and without Down syndrome.

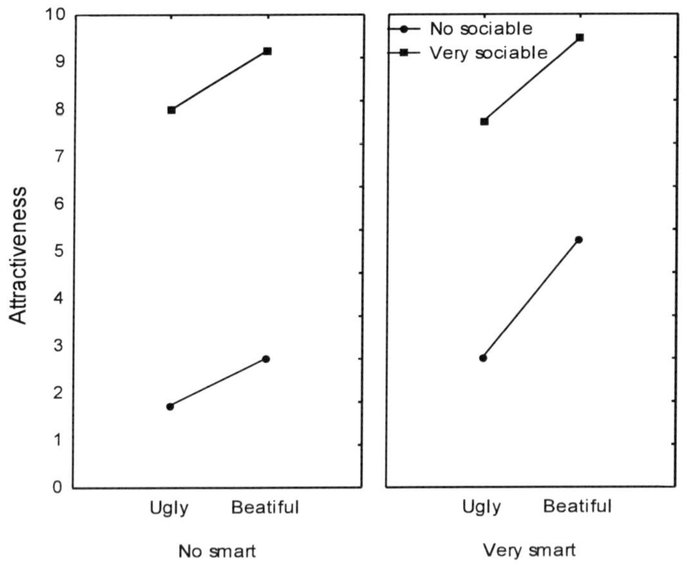

Figure 4.10. These graphs show the interaction effect of Physical appearance, Social personality and Intellectual span on attractiveness judgments for a single participant with Down syndrome (Source: Morales, 2012).

This case is relevant because it reveals the importance of variability inside the same population (DS in this case).

4.4. Some Remarks about the Implications of People with DS' Emotion in Long Term Romantic Relationships

Even when romantic relationships begin by correctly evaluating a potential romantic partner's attributes before formal engagement, the story does not end when a couple is joined (e.g., engagement, marriage, etc.). Romantic partnership evolves through time, and this romantic molding seems to be constrained by a specific, continuous, and dynamic evaluation of the romantic partners' personal attributions. For example, according to Fletcher and Finchman's close relationship attribution model (1991) if a romantic partner has a positive expectancy about a romantic relationship, as well as a positive attitude towards the romantic partner, negative occurrances in the romantic relationship will be attributed to transitory (non-stable) contextual and specific causes (external). On the other hand, positive expectancies about a relationship assume that internal, stable, global good-natured causes are the bases for romantic partner's behaviour inside a close relationship (see Figure 4.9.).

In other words, negative aspects of a close relationship as well as negative attributes to a partner's behaviour are minimized. Simultaneously, positive aspects of a close relationship are maximized. The opposite is true if negative expectancies about a romantic relationship exist (as described by causal attributions in Figure 4.11.). Moreover, in this model attribution it is also assumed that responsibility for a romantic partner's behaviour when in a close relationship is also affected by positive or negative attitudes or expectancies. Thus, the emotional factors of positivity or negativity are extremely important to marital satisfaction. In particular, there is considerable evidence that positive affectivity (Watson, 2000; Watson, Hubbard & Weisee, 2002) as well as negativity (Karney & Bradbury, 1995; Kelly & Conley, 1987) toward a romantic relationship have a significant correlation with marital and relationship satisfaction.

If we frame people with DS' romantic expectancies with theoretical assumptions from the Fletcher and Finchman's close relationship model, we should expect that youth and adults in this population would indeed have a better chance of scoring high on romantic satisfaction tests once they have selected a formal romantic partner (watch a beautiful video on this topic at http://www.monicaanddavid.com). This is suggested by their biased positivity. As a matter of fact, some research suggests that people with ID impose high levels of positivity on their romantic partners and their romantic relationships (Arias, Ovejero & Morentin, 2009).

Now, as it has been pointed through several chapters in this book, people with DS explicitly tend to express positivity. Moreover, academic evidence from Chapter 3 strongly suggests unusually tuned automatic emotion appraisal mechanisms toward positivity. One may wonder how this biased emotional behaviour to positive appraisals affects the youth and adults with DS' most major emotional concern, namely, to be in love.

An initial insight into this concern can be obtained considering love instances inside the DS population. Let us revisit the previously-mentioned video describing the marital life of a couple with DS (Monica and David). According to the close relationship model we just reviewed, and using Monica's "DS emotional eyes", David's "bad marital moments" must be transitory due to some specific misfortune. Instead, she may think he is a great guy (stability and an internal causal attribution) who does well-intentioned things whether these are bad or good things (Unselfishly praised responsibility attributions). The documentary suggests that if specific care is provided to the couple, as well as the opportunity for an independent life (resource accessibility and job opportunities), they will be capable of carrying on a satisfactory marital life. But can they?

Again, there is not sufficient academic research to answer these kinds of questions but certainly the academic exploration we have presented provide examples of possible directions for research in this emotion area. For example IIT research can be implemented to determine if compensatory love schema changes proceed throughout formal romantic relationships of couples with DS, or if memory romantic relational schemata are affected by maximization and minimization of causal and responsibility attributes due to positivity. There is much speculation about the benefits of studying this particular way of experiencing love. Above all concerns is the possibility of improving guidelines to help couples with DS achieve family goals by disassembling a history of beliefs regarding their "difficulties" in comprehending and engaging in formal committed relationships.

So far we have reviewed some aspects of the DS positive emotional system, but it is time to look to another DS definitory attribute, namely, their characteristic way of perceiving and experiencing emotions.

CAUSAL ATTRIBUTIONS

Relationship	Expectancy	INTERNAL	EXTERNAL	STABLE	NON-STABLE	GLOBAL	SPECIFIC
POSITIVE RELATIONSHIP (HAPPY)	POSITIVE EXPECTANCY (CONSISTENT)	•		•		•	
	NEGATIVE EXPECTANCY (INCONSISTENT)		•		•		•
NEGATIVE RELATIONSHIP (UNHAPPY)	POSITIVE EXPECTANCY (INCONSISTENT)		•		•		•
	NEGATIVE EXPECTANCY (CONSISTENT)	•		•		•	

RESPONSIBILITY ATTRIBUTIONS

Relationship	Expectancy	INTENTIONAL	UNINTENTIONAL	SELFISH	UNSELFISH	NO PRAISE	PRAISE	BLAME	NO-BLAME
POSITIVE RELATIONSHIP (HAPPY)	POSITIVE EXPECTANCY (CONSISTENT)	•			•		•		
	NEGATIVE EXPECTANCY (INCONSISTENT)		•		•				•
NEGATIVE RELATIONSHIP (UNHAPPY)	POSITIVE EXPECTANCY (INCONSISTENT)		•	•		•			
	NEGATIVE EXPECTANCY (CONSISTENT)	•		•				•	

Figure 4.11. A model of how positive or negative expectancies in a romantic relationship affect attributions to a romantic partner.

4.5. Down Syndrome and the Negative Emotion Human System

As in the case of positive emotions (e.g., happiness, compassion, love, etc.), negative emotions like hate, resentment, blame, and other negative affectivity deeply define the human condition. The negative range of our emotion spectrum has historically been associated with unpleasant situations, as well as to unfortunate affective experiences, and many research studies on these emotions relate to dysfunctional or pathological emotional behaviour. However, some benefits can be obtained from experiencing negative emotions, even in the most unfavorable situations (see Bastian, Kuppens, Hornsey, Park, Koval, & Uchida, 2012). The emotion of fear facilitates self protection and survival behaviour as well as adaptive responses, blaming someone permits regulatory social interaction, etc. One might wonder how is it that such an important emotional system could be constrained by atypical development, specifically in the case of people with DS, where psychological vulnerability in members of this population is associated with atypical negative emotional development. Let us next introduce some brief academic concerns in this direction.

4.5.1. Down syndrome: the Pain Case

> "Mary (a child with DS) loves to make soap bubbles with her mouth. Even though she knows this makes her sick since every time she does this she gets diarrhea, she always looks forward for an occasion to obtain liquid soap from the kitchen to secretly bubble every place she can."

It is normal to see people look for enjoyable activities, but it is also common to observe that whenever this enjoyment brings more cost than benefit, people desist or abandon the supposedly enjoyable behaviour. Then why is it that many children with DS, like Mary's case described above, will not avoid injurious activities they enjoy? Is this the only result from an inadequately handled behaviour? Or is this misbehaviour strictly related to their genetic condition?

It has been observed that in terms of emotional information processing, most people with people with DS differ from typical ones. Mainly, people with DS tend to have emotion processing limitations over negative valenced information (see Chapters 2 and 3) but there is some variability in the population on this limitation (Morales, 2010). It is unknown if this unique emotional DS characteristic applies to emotional self-perception. For instance, it was only until recently that many considered that people with ID (including people with DS) were insensitive to pain, and that is their pain threshold was very high. However, a research study carried over by Biersdorff (1994) that required family members and caregivers of persons with ID to report their pain responses, observed that at least 52% of the sample with ID showed normal pain responses to averse stimuli. There were also reports of hypersensitivity to pain (11%) and hyposensitivity (37%).

These academic reports help to debunk the "absence of pain attribute" typifying people with ID (see Foley & McCutcheon, 2004). This is relevant to people with DS because they constitute a population with ID with a higher probability of undergoing painful medical interventions, and dismissing the false "painless" attribute helps to avoid unkind treatment (Hennequin, Morin & Feine, 2000).

Nowadays, it is well known that human pain is a multidimensional, complex, subjective experience that includes physical, cognitive and emotional factors that are difficult to explore (Hadjistavropoulos & Craig, 2004; Guneli, Gumustekin, & Ates, 2010). Studying this psychological phenomenon inside the DS population is a real challenge because describing the intensity, severity and localization of a painful sensation is a key component, and language or cognitive limitations often prevent either correct medical intervention or research exploration (Foley & McCutcheon, 2004). To avoid any misconceptions: many people with DS are capable of reporting pain, however, when they have to report localization or explaining the nature or cause of it they tend to be imprecise, and sometimes fail to show the physical expression corresponding to pain (Hennequin, Morin & Feine, 2000).

There are several hypotheses attached to the nature of people with DS' apparent higher pain threshold. Most of these hypotheses include explanatory factors of pain transmission difficulties, problems with integration of pain information, even delayed motor responses (in expressing pain), or a combination of these factors (Hennequin et al., 2000). No doubt, more research about how pain mechanisms behave under the DS genetic condition will bring quality of life improvements over their physical health, and more research is needed in this area., Understanding pain from the psychological side is not an easy matter either.

Multivariate aspects must be considered, and innovative research techniques must be implemented to explore pain. For example, consider the case of psychological pain caused by a friend's transgressive behaviour. The way people with DS use positive or negative information to blame someone who has committed an aggression against them may reveal through blame judgments insights as to how they interpret painful situations. In order to better understand the nature of their possible psychological pain, let us consider the following.

4.6. Moral Emotion and Down Syndrome: Some Academic Remarks on Forgiveness and Blame

"I will never forgive Mike. He hurt me,
What he did to me is unforgiveable....
He is still my friend".

Blame and forgiveness typify many of our life's experiences as humans. We are all constantly exposed to transgressions or we hurt someone else, and thus we feel resentment and are willing to blame others, or to place blame on oneself. On the other hand we have the capacity to forgive and to reconstruct a damaged relationship.

Forgiveness as suggested by its Latin connotation (for/donate) means to give something to someone. To forgive implies to heal emotional wounds, reinstall trust and rebuild a broken relationship (Makinen & Johnson, 2006). There are a variety of motivations behind forgiving (empathy, moral reasons, love, etc.) and granting forgiveness can sometimes be achieved by the presence or even the absence of sincere apologies from the aggressor (Paleari, Regalia & Fincham, 2010), the aggression intentionality (Fein, 2001), the severity of the aggression's consequences (Lopez, 2011), or the personal proximity between the aggressor and the victim (Girard & Mullet, 1997). Some other factors associated with forgiveness are: Victim personality (sympathetic traits; McCullough & Hoyt, 2002), the ability to handle emotions or emotional stability (e.g., Hodgson & Wertheim, 2007), and religiosity (McCullough, Bono, & Root, 2005).

Less known about forgiveness is the impact of atypical development (e.g. DS) on the process. This is a very recent research field. Seminal research on forgiveness and ID can be observed in studies by Roge and Mullet (2011) who introduced the Information Integration theory and its research techniques to exploration of the higher cognitive processing underlying forgiveness and blame inside populations with ID.

Specifically, they presented aggression scenarios to people with autism. Regarding forgiveness, intention and apology factors were considered, whereas scenarios judging blame included intention and consequences. Results from this study showed that even when people with autism used the factor of intention to blame someone in a way similar to that of typical people, they did not weight it in the same way (they valuated it lower). Regarding forgiveness, intention was not considered when judging if an aggressor deserved it or not.

On the same research line, Morales, Charles, Castro, Lopez and Mullet (2012) explored the same cognitive integration information processes inside the DS population. They explored how people with DS systematically integrate (through cognitive algebra) psychologically valuated pieces of information related to blaming (such as intentionality and severity of consequences). To this end, Morales and colleagues (Mullet, Morales, Makris, Rogé & Munoz-Sastre, 2012) adapted the Rogue and Mullets' research instrument (2011) to be used with study samples with DS. Here, scenario aggression contents were converted to auditive stimuli and visual descriptions (comic style). Then the scale was revisualized for the test, and given the title "moral frog" (see Figure 4.12).

As can be observed in Figure 4.12 each scenario describes a transgression that was either intentional or accidental, with consequences that varied in severity (one of: not severe, middle or severe). In total six different situations were considered, containing two levels of intentionality (with and without intention) and three levels of consequences (none, moderate and severe). The participant task was to listen to and watch each vignette and then assign a level of blame to possible aggressor by using the frog's jumps across a scale. Results showed that people with DS are capable of using both pieces of information (intention and consequences) and integrate them through information integration rules, to create blame judgments (see Mullet et al, 2012).

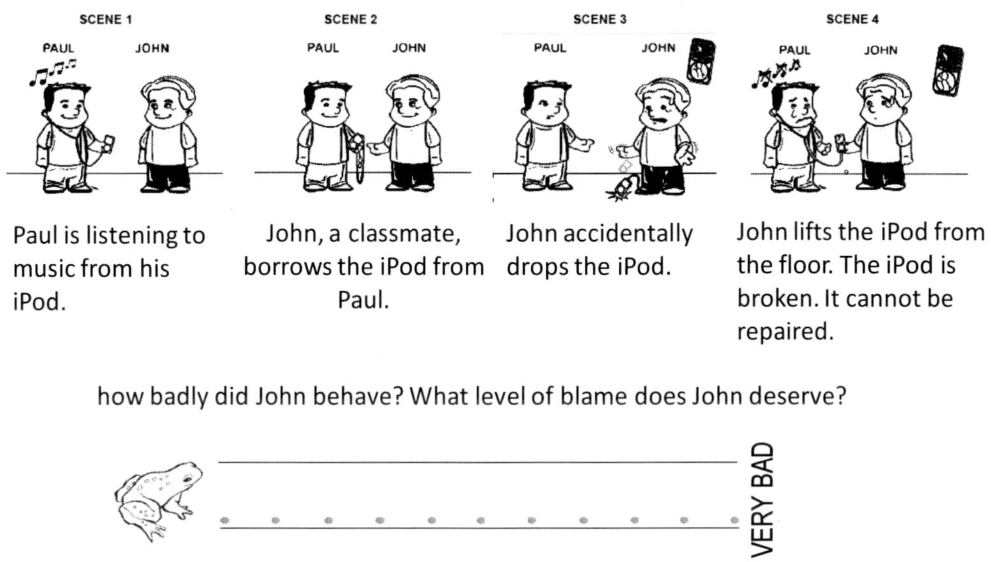

Figure 4.12. An example of a blame scenario from a study carried out by Morales, Charles, Castro, Lopez and Mullet (2012).

A follow up in this line of research (Morales, Lopez & Mullet, 2012) addressed factors of intentionality (accidental or deliberate) as well as an apology factor (no apologies, indirect apologies and direct apologies) to study how people with DS judge, and assign forgiveness. Again, six different aggression scenarios were considered, using the same visual and auditory stimuli, and moral frog scale. Preliminary results showed that in addition to considering apologies as a relevant factor to forgiveness they also consider intention when determining judgment on forgiveness. They use an additive rule to this purpose.

In general, preliminary results from both studies on blame and forgiveness suggest that at least some members of the population with DS are capable of evaluating negative actions, to weigh consequences, and to consider the intentionality of another's behaviour, if they are provided with appropriate contextual information. This capacity to understand how some people may impose pain over other people reveals their capacity for empathy and self-protection, and adaptive social mechanisms to survive inside a social environment that contains many challenges and risks.

4.7. A Brief Summary

As we have argued through this chapter, expanding our understanding of how positive and negative emotion systems develop within atypical developmental conditions could have profound implications on the way people with ID are perceived. It is clear that the presence of DS involves more than a disability. Like many of the rest of us, members of the DS population present strengths and vulnerabilities; these human characteristics frame unique needs to love and to be loved, to search for happiness and even experience moments of sadness. Our point in this chapter has been that academic guidelines provide unique opportunities for improving their lives, either by re-conceptualizing old myths regarding the way they signify their emotional life, or by empowering coping strategies to challenging social environments via emotion education programs.

References

Andersen, S. M., & Cole, S. W. (1990). "Do I know you?": The role of significant others in general social perception. *Journal of Personality and SocialPsychology, 59*, 383-399. Retrieved from http://psycnet.apa.org/index.cfm?fa=buy.optionToBuy&id=1995-40398-001

Anderson, N. H. (1982). *Methods of information integration theory*. New York: Academic Press

Anderson, N. H. (1996). *A functional theory of cognition*. Mahwah, NJ: Erlbaum.

Argyle, M. (2001). *The psychology of happiness* (2nd ed.). New York: Routledge.

Arias, B., Ovejero, A., & Morentin, R., (2009) Love and Emotional Well-being in People with Intellectual Disabilities. *The Spanish Journal of Psychology.12* (1), 204-216.

Baldwin, M. W. &Keelan, J. P. K. (1999). Interpersonal Expectations as a Function of Self-Esteem and Sex. *Journal of Social and Personal Relationships, 16*(6), 822-833. Retrieved from http://selfesteemgames.mcgill.ca/research/baldwinkeelan.pdf

Baldwin, M. W. (1992). Relational schemas and the processing of social information. *Psychological Bulletin, 112,* 461–484. Retrieved from http://selfesteemgames.mcgill.ca/research/baldwnpsybull.pdf

Baldwin, M. W., Fehr, B., Keedian, E., Seidel, M. & Thomson, D. W. (1993). An exploration of the relational schemata underlying attachment styles: Self-report and lexical decision approaches. *Personality and Social Psychology Bulletin, 19*, 746-754. Retrieved from http://www.mcgill.ca/files/social-intelligence/relational_schemata_underlying_attachment.pdf

Baldwin, M. W., Granzberg, A., Pippus, L. & Pritchard, E. T. (2003). Cued activation of relational schemas: Self-evaluation and gender effects. *Canadian Journal of Behavioural Scienc, 35*(2), 153-163. doi: 10.1037/h0087197

Beck, A. T. (1989). *Love Is Never Enough: How Couples Can Overcome Misunderstandings, Resolve Conflicts, and Solve Relationship Problems Through Cognitive Therapy*. Harper Paperbacks.

Capps, L., Kasari, C., Yirmiya, N., & Sigman, M. (1993) Parental perception of emotional expressiveness in children with autism. *J Consult Clin Psychol.61*(3), 475-84. Retrieved from http://psycnet.apa.org/index.cfm?fa=buy.optionToBuy&id=1993-38008-001

Changrian, C. (2010). Happiness and its influencing factors among household heads in urban and rural areas of Thailand. (Doctoral Dissertation, School). Retrieved from http://mng.uru.ac.th/mng/images/present/Sat24854Paper%20at%20Las%20Vegas.pdf

Craddock, N., & Forty, L. (2006). Genetics of affective (mood) disorders. *European Journal of Human Genetics, 14*, 660–668. doi: 10.1038/sj.ejhg.5201549

DeNeve, J. E., Christakis, N.A., Fowler J. H., & Frey, B.S. (2012). Genes, Economics, and Happiness. *Journal of Neuroscience, Psychology, and Economics. 5*(4), 193-211. Retrieved from http://psycnet.apa.org/index.cfm?fa=buy.optionToBuy&id=2012-29455-001

Diener, E. & Diener, C. (1996). Most people are happy. *Psychological Science, 7*, 181-185. doi: 10.1111/j.1467-9280.1996.tb00354.x

Down, J. L. H. (1886) Observations on an Ethnic Classification of Idiots. London Hospital Reports. 259-262

Dykens, E. M., Shah, B., Sagun, J., BeckT. & King, B. H. (2002). Maladaptivebehaviour in children and adolescents withDown's síndrome. *Journal of Intellectual Disability Research, 46*(6), 484-492. doi: 10.1046/j.1365-2788.2002.00431.x

Eastwick, P. W., Finkel, E. J., & Eagly, A.H. (2011). When and why do ideal partner preferences affect the process of initiating and maintaining romantic relationships. *Journal of Personality and Social Psychology, 101*(5), 1012-1032. doi: 10.1037/a0024062

Falconi A. & Mullet, E, (2003). Cognitive Álgebra of love through the adult life. *Intl. J. Again and human development.* 57(3), 275-290.

Farkas, A. J. (1991). Cognitive algebra of interpersonal relationship. In N. H. Anderson (Ed.), *Contributions to information integration theory* (Vol. 2, pp. 43-99). Hillsdale, NJ: Erlbaum.

Fidler, D. J. (2005).The Emerging Down Syndrome Behavioral Phenotype in Early Childhood Implications for Practice. *Infants & Young Children. 18*(2), 86–103. Retrieved from http://depts.washington.edu/isei/iyc/fidler_18_2.pdf

Fidler, D. J., Barrett, K. C. & Most, D. E. (2005). Age-Related Differences in Smiling and Personality in Down Syndrome. *Journal of Developmental and Physical Disabilities, 17*(3), 263-280. doi: 10.1007/s10882-005-4384-x

Fletcher, G. J. O. & Finchman, F. D. (1991). Attribution Processes in Close Relationships. In G. J. O. Fletcher & F. D. Finchman (Eds.), *Cognition in Close Relationships* (pp. 7-31).London: Lawrence Erlbaum Associates.

Fredrickson, B. L. & Cohn, M. A. (2008). Positive emotions. In: Michel Lewis, Jeannette M. Haviland-Jones, & Lisa Feldman Barret (Eds.), *Handbook of Emotions*(3rd ed., pp. 777-796). New York: Guilford Press.

Fredrickson, B. L. (2002). Positive emotions. In: C.R. Snyder, Shane, J. Lopez (Eds.), *Handbook of positive psychology* (pp. 120-134). New York: Oxford University Press.

Fredrickson, B. L. (2005). The broaden-and-build theory of positive emotions. In: F.A. Huppert, N. Baylis, & B. Keverne (Eds.), *The science of well-being*. Oxford, UK: Oxford University Press.pp

Guedj, M., Gibert, M., Maudet, M., Muñoz-Sastre, M. T., Mullet, E. & Sorum, P. C. (2005). The acceptability of ending a patient's life. *J. Med. Ethics, 31*(6), 311-317.

Guedj, M., Muñoz-Sastre, M. T., Mullet, E. & Sorum, P. C. (2009). Is it acceptable for a psychiatrist to break confidentiality to prevent spousal violence? *International Journal of Law and Psychiatry, 32* (2), 108–114.

Guillet, L., Hermand, D. & Mullet, E. (2002). Cognitive processes involved in the appraisal of stress. *Stress and Health, 18*(2), 91–102.

Hendrick, S. S. & Hendrick, C. (1986). A theory and method of love. *Journal of Personality and Social Psychology, 50*, 392-402. Retrieved from http://psycnet.apa.org/index.cfm?fa=buy.optionToBuy&id=1986-13421-001

Hermand, D., Mullet, E., & Lavieville, S. (1997). Perception of the combined effects of smoking and alcohol on cancer risks in never smokers and heavy smokers. *Journal of Health Psychology, 2*(4), 481–491.

Hodapp, R. M. (2001). Etiology and Personality Motivation: Direct and Indirect Effects. In Harvey N. Switzky (Ed.). *Personality and motivational differences in persons with mental* (pp. 247-270). Mahwah, NJ: Lavrrence Erlbaum Associates, Inc.

Hodapp, R. M., Ricci, L. A., Ly, T. M. & Fidler, D. J. (2003). The effects of the child with Down syndrome on maternal stress. *British Journal of Developmental Psychology, 21*, 137–151. doi: 10.1348/026151003321164672

Isen, A. M. (1999). Positive affect. In T. Dalgleish& M.J. Power (Eds.), *Handbook of cognition and emotion* (pp. 521-540). Chichester, UK: Wiley.

Isen, A. M. (2000). Positive affect and decision making. In M. Lewis & J.M. Haviland-Jones (Eds.), Handbook of emotions (2nd ed.). New York: Guilford Press.pp

Isen, A. M. (2008). Some ways in which positive affect influences decision making and problem solving. In: Michel Lewis, Jeannette M. Haviland-Jones, & Lisa Feldman Barret (Eds) *Handbook of Emotions* (3rd ed. pp. 548-573). New York: Guilford Press.

Karney, B. R. & Bradbury, T. N. (1995). The longitudinal course of marital quality and stability: A review of theory, method, and research. *Psychological Bulletin, 118*, 3–34. doi: 10.1037/0033-2909.118.1.3

Kasari, C., Freeman, S. F. & Bass, W. (2003). Empathy and response to distress in children with Down syndrome. *J Child Psychol Psychiatry. 44*(3):424-31. doi: 10.1111/1469-7610.00132

Kelly, E. L. & Conley, J. J. (1987). Personality and compatibility: A prospective analysis of marital stability and marital satisfaction. *Journal of Personality and Social Psychology, 52*, 27-40. doi: 10.1037//0022-3514.52.1.27

Laswell, T. E. & Laswell, M. E. (1976). I love you but I am not in love with you. *Journal of Marriage and the Family*, 38, 211-224. doi: 10.1111/j.1752-0606.1976.tb00413.x

Layard, R. (2005). *Happiness: Lessons from a new science*. London: Penguin.

Lazreg, C. K. & Mullet, E. (2001). Judging the pleasantness of form–color combinations. *The American Journal of Psychology, 114*(4), 511–533.

Lecavalier, L. & Tasse, M. J. (2005). An exploratory study of the ''personality'' of adolescents and adults with Down syndrome. *Journal of Intellectual & Developmental Disability, 30*(2), 67–74. doi: 10.1080/13668250500124976

Lee, J. (1973). *The colors of the love: An exploration of the ways of loving*. Toronto, Canada: New Press.

Lu, L. (2001). Understanding happiness: a look into the Chinese folk psychology. *Journal of Happiness Studies, 2*, 407–432. Retrieved from http://web.ba.ntu.edu.tw/luolu/Understanding%20happiness-A%20look%20into%20the%20Chinese%20folk%20psychology.pdf

Lykken, D. T. (2000). *Happiness.* New York: St. Martin's Griffin.

Lykken, D., & Tellegen, A. (1996). Happiness is a stochastic phenomenon. *Psychological Science,7*(3), 186–189. doi: 10.1111/j.1467-9280.1996.tb00355.x

Lyubomirsky, S. & Lepper, H. S. (1999). A measure of subjective happiness: Preliminary reliability and construct validation. *Social Indicators Research, 46,* 137–155. Retrieved from http://www.psychologytoday.com/files/attachments/496/subjective-happiness-scale.pdf

Lyubomirsky, S. (2007). *The how of happiness: A new approach to getting the life you want.* New York: Penguin Books.

Makri, I. & Mullet, E. (2003). Judging the pleasantness of contour–rhythm–pitch–timbre musical combinations. *The American Journal of Psychology, 116*(4), 581-611.

Morales, G. E. (2012). Functional measurement to cognitive mechanisms underlying attitudes toward sexuality and intellectual disability: New empirical directions. In Nicholas E. Peterson & Whitney Campbell (Eds.), *Sexuality: Perspectives, Issues and Role in Society* (pp. 29- 54). N.Y. USA: Nova Science Publishers, Inc.

Morentin, R., Arias, B., Verdugo, M. A. & Rodriguez-Mayoral, J. M. (2006). Amor y enamoramiento en personas con discapacidad intelectual: un campo por explorar. *Revista española sobre discapacidad intelectual, 37-1*(217), 59-80.

Muñoz-Sastre, M.T., Mullet, E., & Sorum, P.C. (1999). Relationship between cigarette dose and perceived risk of lung cancer. *Preventive Medicine, 28*(6), 566–571.

Murstein, B. I. (1988). A taxonomy of love. En R. J. Sternberg & M. L. Barnes (Eds.), *The psychology of love* (pp. 13-37). New Haven, CT: Yale University Press.

Myers, J. E., Sweeney, T. J. &Witmer, J. M. (2000). The wheel of wellness counseling for wellness: A holistic model for treatment planning. *Journal of Counseling &Development*, 78. 251-266. Retrieved from http://libres.uncg.edu/ir/uncg/f/J_Myers_Wheel_2000.pdf

Neto, F. (1993). Love styles and self representations. *Personality and Individual Differences.*14, 795-803.doi: 10.1016/0191-8869(93)90092-H

Neto, F. (1994). Love styles among Portugese students. *Journal of Psychology, 128*(5), 613-61. doi: 10.1080/00223980.1994.9914919.

Neto, F., & Mullet, E. (1998). Decision making as regards migration: Wage differential, job opportunities and the network effect. *Acta Psychologica, 98*(1), 57-66.

Neto, F., Mullet, E., Deschamps, J., Barros, J., Benvindo, R., Camino, L. & Machado, M. (2000). Cross-Cultural Variations in Attitudes Toward Love. *Journal of Cross-Cultural Psychology*., 31, 5, 626-635. doi: 10.1177/0022022100031005005

Oatley, K. & Jenkins, J. M. (1996). *Understanding emotions*. Cambridge, MA: Blackwell.

Penke, L., Denissen, J. J. A. & Miller, G. F. (2007). The Evolutionary Genetics of Personality. *European Journal of Personality.21*, 549–587. doi: 10.1002/per.629

Pettit, J. W. & Kline, J. P. (2001). Are happy people healthier? The specific role of positive affect in predicting self reported health symptoms. *Journal of Research in Personality, 35*, 521-536. doi: 10.1006/jrpe.2001.2327

Pettit, J. W., Kline, J. P., Gencoz, T., Gencoz, F., & Joiner Jr., T. E. (2001). Are Happy People Healthier? The Specific Role of Positive Affect in Predicting Self-Reported Health Symptoms.*Journal of Research in Personality, 35*(4), 521-536Retrieved from http://home.comcast.nct/~klincjp/pcttit.pdf

Power, M. & Dalgleish, T. (2008). *Cognition and Emotion: From order to disorder* (2nd ed.). Hove: Psychology Press.

Reeder, H. M. (1996). The subjective experience of love through the adult life. *International Journal of Aging and Human Development, 43,* 325-340. doi: 10.2190/V7J3-XQAL-2X59-M16X

Robison, R. J. (2000). Learning About Happiness From Persons With Down Syndrome: Feeling the Sense of Joy and Contentment. *American journal on Mental Retardation,105*(5), 372-376. doi: 10.1352/0895-8017(2000)105<0372:LAHFPW> 2.0.CO;2

Schwartz, R. M. (1992). States of mind model and personal construct theory: Implications for psychopathology. *International Journal of Personal Construct Psychology, 5*, 123–143. doi: 10.1080/08936039208404306

Shaver, P. R., Wu, S. & Schwartz, J. C. (1992). Cross-cultural similarities and differences in emotion and its representation: A prototype approach. In M.S. Clark (Ed.), *Review of personality and social psychology* (Vol. 13, pp. 175-212). Newbury Park, CA: Sage.

Simpson, J. A. & Gangestad, S. W. (1992). Socio-sexuality and romantic partner choice. *Journal of Personality, 60*, 31–51. Retrieved from http://ablongman.com/partners _in_psych/PDFs/Kenrick/kenrick_CH10.pdf

Skotko, B. G, Levine, S. P., & Goldstein, R. (2011). Self-Perceptions from People with Down syndrome. *American Journal of Medical Genetics, 155*, 2360-2369. doi: 10.1002/ ajmg.a.34235

Stein M. B, Campbell-Sills L. & Gelernter, J. (2009). Genetic Variation in 5HTTLPR Is Associated With Emotional Resilience. *Am J Med Genet B NeuropsychiatrGenet.150B(7) 900–906.* doi: 10.1002/ajmg.b.30916.

Sternberg, R. J. (1986). A triangular theory of love. *Psychological Review*, 93, 119-135. doi: 10.1037/0033-295X.93.2.119

Sternberg, R. J. (1988). Triangulating love. In R.J. Sternberg & M.L. Barnes (Eds.), *The psychology of love* (pp. 119-138). New Haven, CT: Yale University Press.

Sternberg, R. J. (1997). Construct validation of a triangular love scale.*European Journal of Social Psychology*, 27, 313-335. doi: 10.1002/(SICI)1099-0992(199705)27:3<313::AID-EJSP824>3.0.CO;2-4

Tallis, F. (2004). *Love sick: Love as a mental illness*. London: Century.

United Nations. (2012). *World Happiness Report*.The earth institute, Columbia University.Retrieved from http://www.earth.columbia.edu/sitefiles/file/Sachs%20 Writing/2012/World%20Happiness%20Report.pdf

Veenhoven, R. (1984). Conditions of happiness. Dordrecht, The Netherlands: D. Reidel.*Abstract retrieved fromhttp://www2.eur.nl/fsw/research/veenhoven/Pub1980s/ 84a2-ab.htm*

Veenhoven, R. (1991). Is happiness relative? *Social Indicators Research 24*,1 –34. Retrieved from http://www2.eur.nl/fsw/research/veenhoven/Pub1990s/91a-full.pdf

Watson, D. (2002). Positive affectivity: The disposition to experience pleasurable emotional States. In: C.R. Snyder, Shane, J. Lopez (Eds.), *Handbook of positive psychology* (pp. 106-119). New York: Oxford University Press.

Watson, D., Hubbard, B. & Wiese, D. (2000). General traits of personality and affectivity as predictors of satisfaction in intimate relationships: Evidence from self- and partner-ratings. *Journal of Personality, 68*(3), 413–449. doi: 10.1111/1467-6494.00102

Weinberg, R. A. (1989). Intelligence and IQ: Landmark issues and great debates. *American Psychologist, 44*, 98–104. doi: 10.1037/0003-066X.44.2.98

Wishart, J. G. & Johnston, F. H. (1990).The effects of experience on attribution of a stereotyped personality to children with Down's syndrome.*Journal of Mental Deficiency Research, 34*(5), 409-420.

Wuang, Y. P. & Su, C. Y. (2012). Patterns of participation and enjoyment in adolescents with Down syndrome. *Research in Developmental Disabilities, 33*(3), 841–848. doi: http://dx.doi.org/10.1016/j.ridd.2011.12.008

Chapter 5

Future Directions in the Study of the Down Syndrome's Emotional World

Abstract

People with DS are a minority group that has to overcome many obstacles to get a job, a dignified life or being considered by the community as a participant (Werner, Corrigan, Ditchman & Sokol, 2012). As a matter of fact, for a long time their human rights were not acknowledged nor even considered (Morales, 2013). A variety of factors have contributed to this stigma. For example, it is common to reduce the whole person to a single characteristic, that is, a genetic condition named Down syndrome. This biological constraint has created and fostered a system of misbeliefs and mischaracterisations that not only impose many limitations to members of this populations but also upon parents and caregivers dealing with DS.

As we have been suggesting elsewhere in this book, current scientific understanding about people with DS can be used to dismantle or demystify outdated beliefs about DS intellectual and behavioural manifestations. No doubt that initial inquiries about the way people with DS signify and emotionally experience life bring up more questions about their psychological perceptions. By better understanding this psychological diversity we empower institutions and people dealing with this syndrome to provide improvements over the quality of their lives. To this end, let us reconsider the current academic status on emotion and DS as well as some new research trends in this direction inside human emotion theory research.

5.1. General Remarks about Emotion Research Regarding People with Down Syndrome

Academic scrutiny on DS emotional system has recently begun, though in contrast to other emotion research dealing with intellectual disability there are as yet too few research publications. This makes difficult to characterize the emotional lives of people having this syndrome. Indeed, most clinical approaches, as well as educational strategies dealing with peoples with DS' emotional life, are based on other ID population characteristics. Even when the two populations share several cognitive and behavioural abilities, these communalities do not imply equivalence and by no means can an equivalence be made between the entire DS cognitive-emotional frame and populations with other IDs. Consequently, two immediate and obvious demands emerge: First, more empirical research on emotion and DS such as are presented in this book is needed. Second, as suggested by the National Disability Authority (2002a, b), people with DS must not only be allowed to participate in academic research but they should also be encouraged to do so when this academic research is related to improvements over their life quality. This guarantees an inclusive vision over factors that are relevant to members of this population.

In order to be compliant with with this research view one might consider factors like a) their complex emotional nature, b) their inherent definitory population characteristics, c) and d) the existing methodological and theoretical development inside the field.

In terms of the DS emotional nature, we have already introduced some academic remarks as well as some suggestion for future research, however, additional considerations can be obtained from Points b, c, and d in the following section.

5.1.1. Research Considerations on Sample with DS Inherent Characteristics

There are many research challenges whenever samples with DS are considered in studies of emotion. First, historical factors typify this population as extremely vulnerable to non ethical intentions (Edwards, 2000), and many are afraid they could be exploited, or abused as has happened in the past in other research fields (e.g. the Willowbrook experiments: Iacono, 2006; Nazi medical practices: McClimens & Allmark, 2011). Because of these unethical approaches in the past to academic research, it is understandable why nowadays parents, teachers and caregivers related to ID are not inclined to consider active participation in academic research. Here, sensitivity, humane and well-intentioned research are initial steps to sample inclusion. Some simple strategies to this purpose are:

- Practice listening to study participants' concerns, as well as to any information from parents or people who are responsible for their security.
- Take your time in describing the possible short, middle and long term gains to this population when talking to participants, parents, teachers, etc. about the benefits.
- Respect the biological and psychological necessities of potential study participants, and remember they are allowing us to enter inside their lives.

Some other simple and logical considerations can be presented (which are frequently forgotten by researchers) to convince participants with ID to participate in scientific research. In our experience it is complete respect for their human condition rather than just to their syndrome that convinces people with DS and their relatives, teachers, etc., to participate in scientific research. This in turn helps researchers to avoid any complications with their experimental design.

On the other hand, do not forget to consider inherent DS cognitive constraints when recruiting members of this population. This is a population characterized by a wide set of cognitive abilities (Tsao & Kindelberger, 2009; Edwards, 2000). This variability makes it difficult to provide the same participation rank to every person with DS and researchers must be carefully about possible effects on their results due to this. Here, if no exact acknowledgment of cognitive functioning for every participant is achieved, then sample inclusion should concentrate over those participants with higher cognitive performance (McClimens & Allmark, 2011).

a) Theoretical Development

Since models or paradigms based on the concept of sickness (e.g. rehabilitation or medical models) have permeated the psychological study of intellectual disability, most research in this field has been carried out applying the concepts of loss or deficits. Furthermore, the psychological concept of normality has had a profound impact over research trends inside the ID field. For instance, not long ago, concepts like "subnormal" or "non normal" were inappropriately used to define intellectual disability. These conceptualizations have been central in maintaining a system of misbeliefs and stigmas attached to this population (Morales, 2013). No doubt that better theoretical accounts other than the "deficit" concept are needed to really understand the person living with a genetic constrained emotional system

It is encouraging to observe a growing number of persons interested on understanding people with DS' human necessities. Take for instance that nowadays people in or connected with this population are willing to talk about topics that were supposedly exclusive to typical people's concerns. Discussions about DS and love or emotional disorders like depression and DS can be found on the Internet. These kinds of discussions were not even considered a possibility in the past, and the goal now is to maintain this interest by providing new scientific insights over the human conditions within DS.

A recent review of different academic digital bases (Psychology and Behavioral Sciences Collection, Academic Search Complete, Education Research Complete, ERIC, MEDLINE, Professional Development Collection, PsycARTICLES, PsycINFO, SocINDEX with Full Text, eBook Collection) using combination of words like emotion, intellectual disability, mental retardation, and Down syndrome resulted in 425 papers, of which only 39 were related to emotion research and DS (direct measurement). Figure 5.1. graphically shows the range of emotion topics considered in this last category.

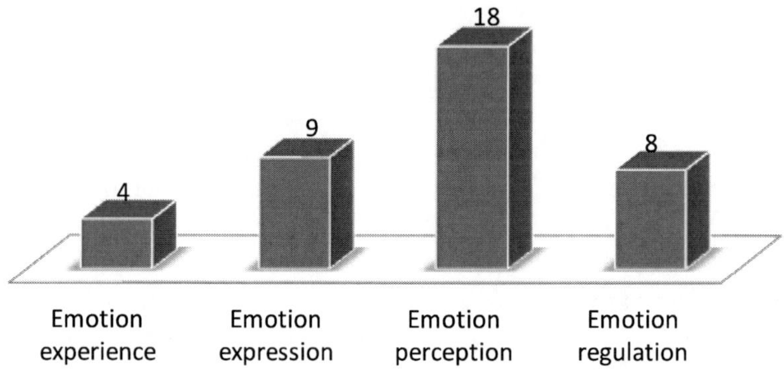

Figure 5.1. Number of published scientific papers on DS and different emotions between the years 2000 and 2011.

Each of these emotion topics (see table 1) encompasses a range of psychological phenomena from central information processing (e.g., schemata activation, social scripts, inference, etc) to peripheral information processing (e.g. face emotion recognition).

Table 5.1. Emotion topics distribution over four possible emotional dimensions

Emotional dimension	Topic	Number of papers
Emotion experience	Motivation	1
	Empathy	1
	Friendship	2
Emotion expression	Humour	2
	Emotional development	1
	Facial expression	1
	Emotional responses	1
	Emotional development	1
	Affective expression	3
Emotion perception	Facial emotion processing	9
	Friendship	1
	Emotional processing	1
	Emotional attribution	1
	Emotion interaction	1
	Facial and vocal emotion processing	1
	Emotional development	1
	Effects of emotion profile on socio-cognitive behaviour	1
	Self-Perceptions	1
	Pain	1
Emotion regulation	Effects of mood on behaviour	1
	Effects of emotion profile on socio-cognitive behaviour	2
	Emotional competence	1
	Emotional aspect of Temperament	1
	Affective expression	1
	Emotional development	1
	Emotional responses	1
		39

Note in both Figure 1 and Table 1 that most research papers relate to emotion perception. An interesting fact about these papers is that more than 50% of them deal with face emotion recognition. Unfortunately, no theoretical considerations for models relating emotion and DS were found in these database searches.

Overall this digital academic search suggests that three lines of research have predominated emotion and DS:

1. People with DS's development and experience of emotion: This study area is concerned with emotion regulation, the way emotion is experienced, and it mainly

uses indirect sources of information to academic research (e.g. parents, teachers, caregivers, etc.) (See Chapters 2, 3, 4).

2. The way people with DS perceive their own emotion: Here, academic scrutiny concentrates on the way members of this population acknowledge and make attributions regarding their emotional lives (see Chapter 4).
3. The way other people (e.g. parents, teachers, caregivers, etc.) perceive people with DS's emotional life: This research area regards other people's attributions and knowledge of the emotional life of people with DS (e.g., Humor, Reddy, Williams & Vaughan, 2002; Reddy, Williams, & Vaughan, 2001; temperament, Nygaard, Smith & Torgersen, 2002).

As may be recognized, this book has been concerned with point 1 (People with DS's development and experience of emotion) and point 2 (People with DS's self perception of emotion). We strongly believe this overview encourages new research trend lines to include human and psychological peculiarities of this population into human emotion theory.

b) Methodological Development

Although scientific analysis of human emotion has recently begun, there has already been time to develop a wide set of research instruments and methods to study it. Looking at the last decade of DS study, there has been an increasing academic interest in developing scaling methods, implementing standardized and non-standardized emotional face recognition tasks (e.g., Facial recognition tests, Christensen, Riley, Heffernan, Love & MacLaughlin, 2002; facial emotion categorization tasks, Leder, Schwarzer & Langton, 2003; the preferential-looking technique, Mondloch, 1999), development of experimental tasks (e.g., affective priming, Fazio, 2001), and other research techniques in order to explore the development of emotion, and the way emotion is experienced and perceived by members of this population (see Figure 5.2).

Methodological developments have been mainly focused on finding common behavioural and psychological patterns inside this population in order to typify them and look for intervention programs (clinical and educative). However, bear in mind what this book proposes is an emphasis rather on developing research instruments to study diversity, especially whenever DS emotion is considered.

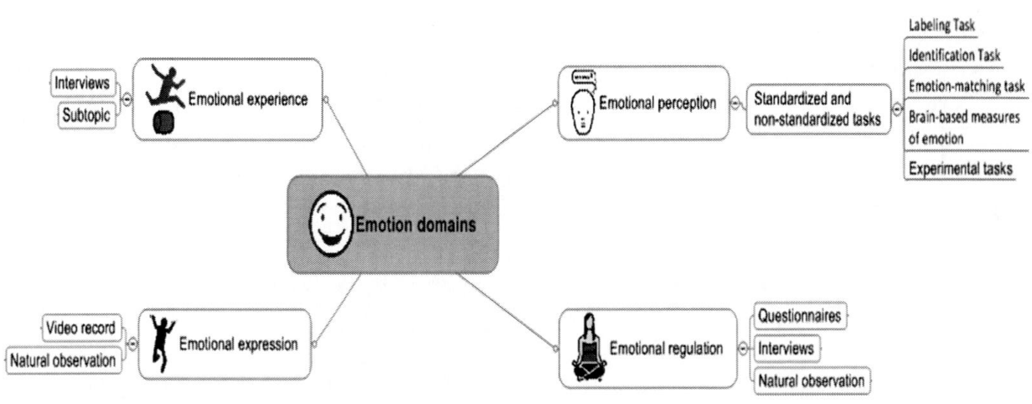

Figure 5.2. Some research instruments used to study emotion and DS.

5.2. Future Possible Research Trends in Emotion and DS

In terms of emotion and DS we have only considered in this book a relatively few topics (e.g. Love, happiness, forgiveness, hate, blame, etc.). By no means has research to date in these emotion processes revealed all the emotional complexity of a person with DS, and much more research is needed. However, have in mind that a strong emphasis has been made through this book on considering ecological validity whenever research is conducted on emotion and DS. Whether you are considering the way someone with DS expresses or recognizes emotion faces, or how negativity is processed within social contexts, the previously described academic research suggests that it is always necessary to consider stimuli relevant to this population. For example, using DS faces in a face recognition experiment, or testing using social situations relevant to cognitive ruled information integration (e.g. framed by DS positivity or limitations on processing negative information). At the end we strongly suggest that possible future directions on emotion and DS should address *the human condition* and not *the genetic condition* or *the intellectual disability* typifying this population.

In this spirit, the algebra cognitive technique considered (Chapter 4) allows introduction of everyday situations framed by DS emotional considerations, and at the same time provides a powerful analysis of higher cognitive processing participation over such social scenarios. This is also the case for affective priming research and emotion face recognition. Complex experimental designs with easy emotion identification tasks suitable to DS' emotional abilities, empowers theoretical development on emotion and DS. This is also true for emotion categorization tasks considered on when defining Russells' emotion circumplex. Overall, these research methods offer an invitation to deepen our understanding beyond the current academic status on emotion and DS, and thus foster positive impact of academic guidelines over the quality of life in this population.

5.3. Telling the Story in a Nutshell

Science offers a window into a human condition that is typified by a particular way of expressing, experiencing, and signifying emotion. Through these chapters we have considered a diversity of uncommon research methods inside the study of intellectual disabilities and the variety of emotion topics relevant people with DS's emotional life (Figure 5.3). In particular, we have discussed how initial academic research on DS was implicitly geared toward a negative conceptualization of human variability (Chapter 1). This negative impression had a profound effect on people with DS's quality of life since this genetic variation was conceptualized as a sickness or deficit and not as a life condition.

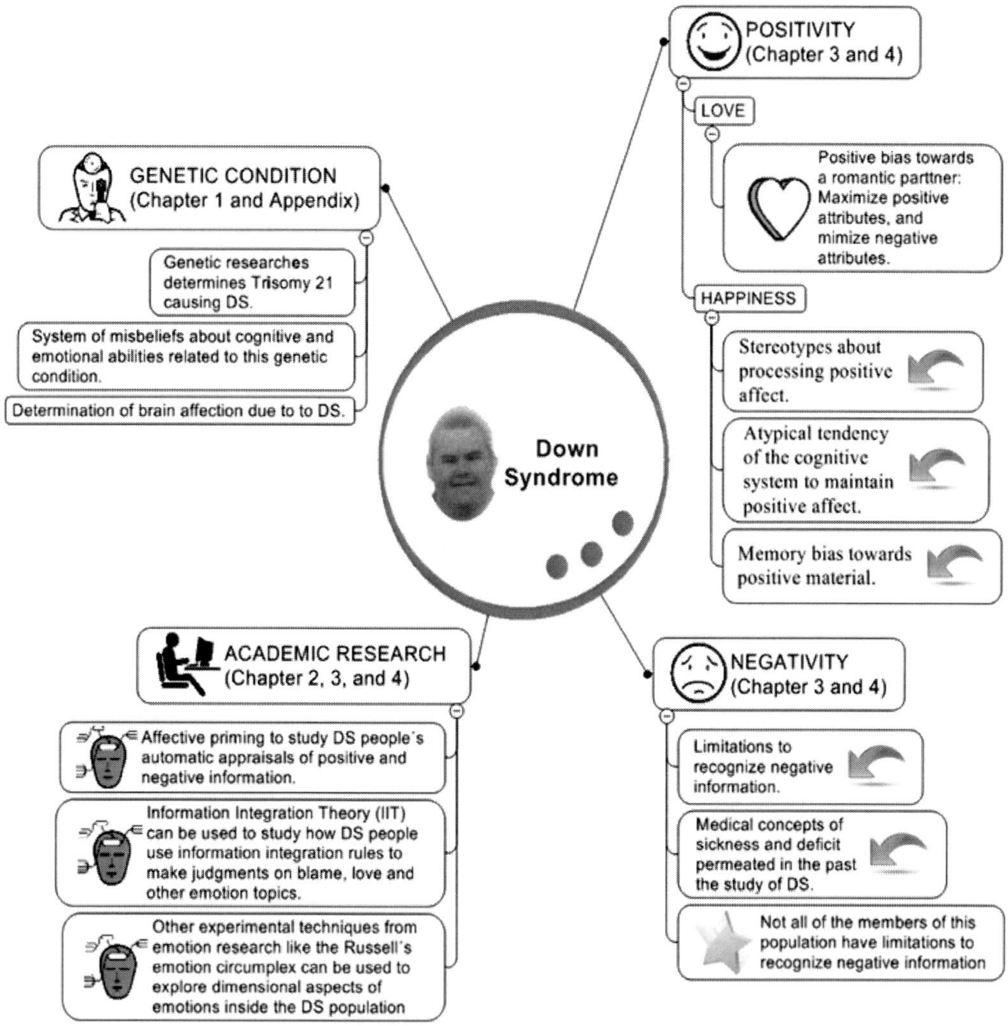

Figure 5.3. A visual representation of some of the book's main points.

Historically, we have struggled to understand what human variability means. By considering the way people with DS express and experience emotion we have argued over how nature can find another way to consciously signify life through emotion. In turn this alternative way of emotionally experiencing life provides more insightful ideas about who we are. Ongoing academic interest regarding the instances in which biological organisms experience emotion, will certainly lead to the establishment of a set of principles of emotional behaviour. Moreover, we will have a better understanding of the emotional similarities and differences among different groups of our own species (including DS). To this end we have introduced in this book some experimental approaches empowering scientific analysis on emotion and DS (perception, expression, experience and emotional regulation; see chapter 2). For instance by considering affective priming research we have discussed unique characteristics typifying people with DS's automatic processing bias and processing limitations of negative and positive information (chapter 3). In short this academic scrutiny suggests that not all people with DS process negative information the same way, that most study participants with DS showed a strong bias toward processing positive information—similar in some instances to typical individuals' preferences toward positivity. Most interesting was the observation of a remarkable bias toward process familiar emotion faces (DS faces).

However, regarding the DS processing mechanisms of positive information, it's fair to say that this cognitive-emotional system remains almost a complete mystery and that more research is needed. Considering for instance our discussion on love and happiness from Chapter 4, there is no doubt that these emotional topics are a major concern for people with DS when coping with daily problems, and yet we know too little about them, especially if our level of understanding is compared with what we know about these emotional dimensions inside a typical population.

Academic remarks have been presented in this book which consider the human necessity of people with DS to have romantic relationships and to experience love. This proposal is supported by cognitive algebra studies in Chapter 4 showing that even considering that they valuate potential romantic partner's attributes in a different way from that of a typical person, they use similar higher cognitive processing in selecting someone to love (e.g. using the same information integration rule). This higher cognitive processing also seems to be present in other mental activity (e.g. assigning blame).

The intention of this book is not to be a set of guidelines to be dogmatically adhered to when considering the way people with DS feel and emotionally signify their lives. Rather, academic considerations of a diversity of emotion topics have been discussed as an invitation to explore new empirical directions, in order to push forward the current academic knowledge and understanding of emotion and DS. Research tools are now available for this purpose and we are on the verge of an academic breakthrough.

References

Christensen, K. J., Riley, B. E., Heffernan, K. A., Love, S. B., & MacLaughlin Sta. Maria, M. E. (2002). Facial recognition test in the elderly: norms, reliability and premorbid estimation. 16 (1), 51-56.

Edwards S. D. (2000). An argument against research on people with intellectual disabilities. *Medicine, Health Care, And Philosophy, 3*(1), 69-73.

Fazio, R. H. (2001). On the automatic activation of associated evaluations: An overview. *Cognition & Emotion, 15*(2), 115-141. doi: 10.1080/0269993004200024.

Iacono, T. (2006). Ethical challenges and complexities of including people with intellectual disability as participants in research. *Journal of Intellectual & Developmental Disability, 31*(3), 173-179.

Leder, H., Schwarzer, G. y Langton, S. (2003). Development of face processing in early adolescence. In G. Schwarzer, y H. Leder, The development of face processing (págs. 69-80). USA: Hogrefe y Huber Publishers.

McClimens, A. & Allmark, P. (2011). A problem with inclusion in learning disability research. *Nursing Ethics, 18*(5), 633-639.

Mondloch, C.J., Lewis, T. L., Budreau, D. R.,Murer, D., Dannemiller, J. L., Stephens, B. R. y Kleiner-Gathercoal, K. A. (1999). Face percepetion during early infancy. *Psychological Science, 10*(5), 419-422.

Morales, G. E., Lopez, E.O., Charles, D. J., Castro, C. & Sanchez, M. P. (2013). Parental and Educators' Judgments and Attitudes toward Life Challenges of people with Intellectual Disability: Functional Measurement Contributions to Special Education from a Cognitive Algebra Approach. In A. Thurgood and K. Schuldt (Eds.). *Caregivers: Challenges, Practices and Cultural Influences*. N.Y. USA: Nova Publisher.

National Disability Authority (2002a). *Guidelines for Including People with Disabilities in Research*. National Disability Authority, Dublin, Ireland.

National Disability Authority (2002b). *Ask Me: Guidelines for Effective Consultation with People with Disabilities*. National Disability Authority, Dublin.

Nygaard, E., Smith, L. & Torgersen, A. M. (2002).Temperament in children with Down syndrome and in prematurely born children. *Scandinavian Journal of psychology, 43*, 61-71

Reddy, V., Williams, E. & Vaughan, A. (2002). Sharing humour and laughter in autism and Down's syndrome. *British Journal Psychology, 93*, 219-242.

Reddy, V., Williams, E. & Vaughan, A. (2001). Sharing laughter: the humor of pre-school children with Down syndrome. *Down syndrome research and Practice, 7*(3), 125-128.

Tsao, R. & Kindelberger, C. (2009). Variability of cognitive development in children with Down syndrome: Relevance of good reasons for using the cluster procedure. Research in Developmental Disabilities, 30(3), 426-432.doi: 10.1016/j.ridd.2008.10.009.

Werner S Corrigan P, Ditchman N. & Sokol K. (2012). Stigma and intellectual disability: a review of related measures and future directions. *Research in Developmental Disabilities, 33*(2),748-65. doi: 10.1016/j.ridd.2011.10.009.

Appendix A

Nowadays, a noticeable growing interest on DS in different academic fields can be observed. One motivation underlying this attention is that this genetic condition comprises a third part of intellectual disability cases (Hodapp, DesJardín & Ricci, 2003; Paterson & Costa, 2005). In addition, life expectancy in this population has been increasing thus demanding more understanding about the way in which members of this population are participants in society, and their social concerns (cognitive competency, labor concerns, social emotions, lifespan development, education, etc.). No doubt that a major advance in understanding DS was the discovery of the genetic mechanism underlying this condition by Dr. Lejuene in 1959. Let us discuss more on DS genetic mechanisms next.

The Same Origin but Different Paths

Engendering a new human being begins with a process called fecundation. Here, the feminine and masculine gametes (sexual cells) join together to create the zygote (or fertilized ovum cell) (see Figure A.1). After this union, a process named mitosis begins. This refers to the process where the zygote duplicates itself until a new pluricellular organism is formed. This kind of cellular division occurs only in non sexual cells or somatic cells and continues throughout our lives, with our old cells replaced by new cells (Langman, 1981; Parker & Kolthoff, 1977).

Before fertilization, germinative cells tend to experience chages through a process called "meiosis" (I, and II). These transformations allow the spermatozoon to provide only 23 chromosomes and the ovule provide the other 23 chromosomes such that the new organisms will contain 46 chromosmes. This is the number of chromosomes a typical human being has in each cell. However, this is not always the case. A person may be born with less (Autosomy: one less chromosome) or more chromosomes (Trysomy: Whenever there are three chromosomes instead of two in any chromosomal pair). People with Down syndrome are born with an additional chromosome number 21, that is, they have three chromosome 21. It is for this reason that DS is also known as Trisomy 21 (it is not coincidence that the 21st day of the third month of every year is World Down Syndrome Day). In short, every person with DSis born with 47 chromosomes. How is this possible?

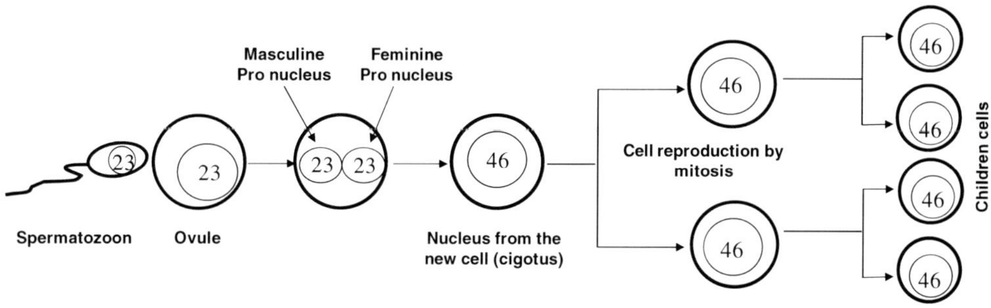

Figura A.1. Fecundation: The spermatozoon and the ovule provide 23 chromosomes each engender a new unicellular organism, the zygote (cigotus). After the engendered cell is achieved through mitosis it becomes a pluricellular organism.

Well, the regular Trisomy 21 occurs as result of a distribution error, generally during the female/male's sexual cell production (spermatozoids or ovules). More specifically, during meiotic division, either the spermatozoid or the ovule contributes an extra chromosome 21 (Figure A.2.). Most frequently it is the ovule that makes this contribution causes all of that child's cells to contain three 21 chromosomes instead of two (Jasso, 1991; Lambert & Rondal, 1989; Stratford, 1998).

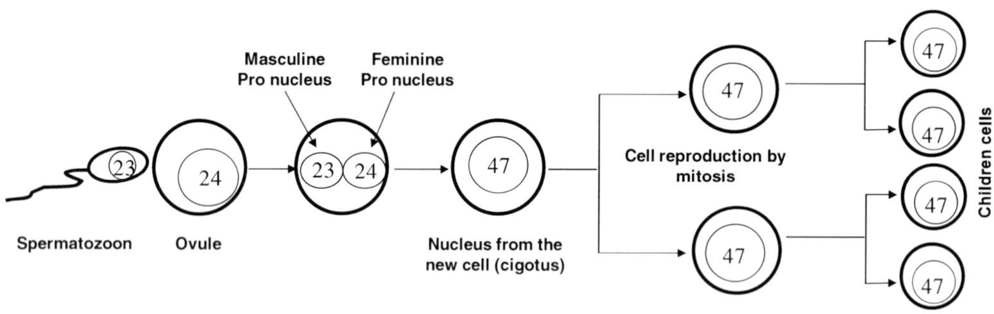

Figure A.2. An example of regular trisomy 21.

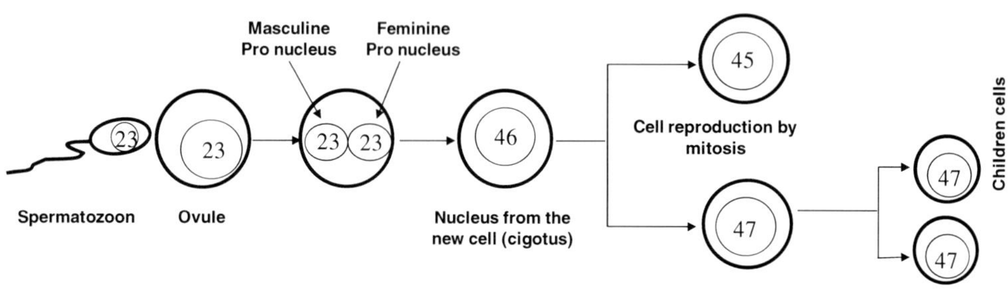

Figura A.3. Trisomy 21 as the result of chromosome distribution error in the first cellular division.

As can be seen from Figure A.2., another possible genetic DS scenario is when a sexual cell contributes an additional chromosome 21 during fecundation, provide as a result a new cell with three 21 chromosomes. As a consequence, all the child's cells will have trisomy.

Alternatively, a chromosome with no disjunction (neither of the chromosomes 21 separate adquately) during the first cellular division after fecundation also produces trisomy

21 (Jasso, 1991). Thus all of the organism's cells will have the same genetic condition (Figure A.3.)

Another genetic process that leads to DS is known as Mosaicism. In this case, trisomy 21 occurs either at the time or after the second cell division that follows fecundation (Figure A.4.).

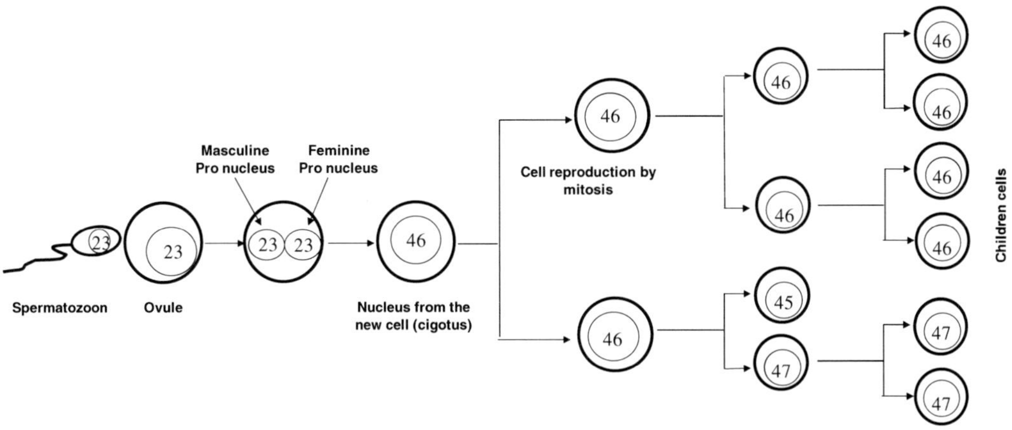

Figure A.4. Graphic display showing chromosome distribution error when a second cellular division occurs after fecundation. Some portion of the cells will posses 47 chromosomes and some will only have 46. This genetic constrained condition is known as mosaic DS.

A third genetic process leading to DS is named translocation. In this case chomosome 21, or part of it, is blended or translocates to another chromosome (e.g., 14, 22).

As a final comment, have in mind that no matter which genetic process underlies DS acquisition, people with this syndrome are complete human beings having desires and life aspirations. Their ability to live a full life depends on the support our society provides.

References

Hodapp, R., DesJardín, J. & Ricci, L. (2003). Genetic Syndromes of Mental Retardation: Should they matter for the early interventionist? *Infants and Young Children*, 16(2), 152-160.

Jasso, L. (1991). *El niños Down: mitos y realidades.* México, D.F.: Manual moderno.

Lagman, J. (1981). *Embriología Médica*. México: Médica Panamericana.

Lambert, J. & Rondal, J. (1989). *El mongolismo.* Barcelona: Herder.

Patterson, D. & Costa, A. C. S. (2005). History of genetic disease: Down syndrome and genetics a case of linked histories. *Nature Reviews Genetics*,6, 137-147.

Parker, C. & Kolthoff, N. (1977). *Anatomía y Fisiología*. México: Nueva Editorial Interamericana.

Stratford, B. (1998). *Síndrome de Down: Pasado, presente y futuro*. México: Edivision.

Subject Index

Author Index

V

W

Y

Z